the
dairy-
free
detox diet

Also available from Thorsons

By Dawn Hamilton (with Antoinette Savill):
Lose Wheat, Lose Weight
Super Energy Detox

By Jane Sen:
Eat to Beat Cancer (with Dr Rosy Daniel)
Healing Foods Cookbook
More Healing Foods

the
dairy-
free
detox diet

Dawn Hamilton, Ph.D.

with recipes by Jane Sen

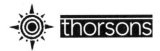

Thorsons
An Imprint of HarperCollins*Publishers*
77–85 Fulham Palace Road,
Hammersmith, London W6 8JB

The website address is: www.thorsonselement.com

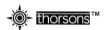

and *Thorsons* are trademarks of
HarperCollins*Publishers* Ltd

Published by Thorsons 2003

10 9 8 7 6 5 4 3 2 1

A catalogue record of this book is
available from the British Library

ISBN 0 00 714787 2

Printed and bound in Great Britain by
Creative Print and Design (Wales), Ebbw Vale

contents

1: the dairy-free detox diet

Like many of us, Robert loves ice cream. But he doesn't eat it very often because of the effect this food has on his health. Within an hour of eating it he starts wheezing, has difficulty breathing and suffers with a blocked nose. This reaction usually lasts for several hours until his respiratory system returns to normal.

Robert's case is typical of many people who have an intolerance to dairy foods. He has never suffered with asthma and his respiratory system is perfectly healthy – except when he consumes dairy. As Robert eats dairy foods only once or twice a year, the effects on his health are very visible. However, it's easy to overlook the link between dairy and our health if we consume dairy foods on a regular basis. We may suffer from annoying, uncomfortable and distressing health conditions without realizing the cause may be found in our diet. These symptoms can be physical or mental, including:

- a blocked nose
- digestive problems
- fluid retention
- poor skin
- an inability to concentrate
- feeling tired all of the time
- emotional ups and downs
- depression

We may just assume that these symptoms are simply part and parcel of life. We put them down to stress, getting older or simply working too hard. But the reality is that **having a food intolerance problem can place a big toll on our overall health and wellbeing. We may feel that our 'get up and go' has definitely got up and gone or that the sparkle of life has disappeared.** Yet when the offending foods are removed from the diet for a period of time and steps are taken to strengthen the body systems involved in intolerance, there is often a big improvement in how we feel and how we look.

about this book

This book will help you find out whether or not you have an intolerance to dairy products. It offers you a range of nutritional strategies to help regain your lost vitality and health. You will also find out how to create a really healthy, dairy-free diet that's tailor-made to your own needs. These guiding principles should help keep you in good health for years to come.

The first few chapters of this book explain what dairy intolerance is and how it can develop. You might have heard the term 'lactose intolerance' but dairy intolerance is something quite different. The difference between these two conditions is described in Chapters 2 and 3, and Chapter 4 discusses other aspects of the relationship between dairy and our health, such as the link with certain serious diseases.

In Chapter 5 you will read about a simple yet highly effective dietary principle that can have a fantastically positive impact on our energy levels, mood and overall health. Chapters 6 through 12 outline the programme itself. Everything you need to do to find out whether you are genuinely intolerant to dairy is outlined in clear and easy steps. Foods to eat and those to avoid are described in Chapter 7.

Our diet can have a tremendous impact on our health. Different foods can be either harming or healing for the body. In Chapter 8, you will read about specific 'superfoods' that have natural healing qualities and can help you overcome health symptoms associated with dairy intolerance.

In addition, there are several other nutritional strategies for you to try that will help strengthen the physical systems usually involved with food intolerance. These include steps to improve the health of your digestive system and natural ways of supporting your hard-working liver.

Later chapters take a more long-term view. Chapter 11 explains why certain dietary fats are vital to our health. While we all need these essential fats, they are particularly important for people who have a dairy intolerance as they are often unable to utilize these fats properly. This is especially true in cases of eczema, poor skin and premenstrual syndrome. Having a food intolerance problem can make it difficult to lose weight, even when following a calorie-controlled diet. So Chapter 12 explores the relationship between food intolerance and weight loss and offers you a number of strategies that can help you achieve healthy and permanent weight loss without calorie counting or ever feeling really hungry.

Chapter 13 shows you how to make sure you are meeting your calcium needs and, importantly, how to balance your calcium intake with other essential nutrients. Keeping your bones healthy requires much more than just getting adequate calcium. There are lots of dietary and lifestyle factors that can have a negative effect on the health of your bones. Chapter 14 outlines what these factors are so that you can take steps to keep your bones strong throughout your life. Chapter 15 looks at the problems with modern dairy farming. Chapter 16 gives further information on the science behind the dietary advice.

Did You Know?

If you do have a dairy intolerance, you should expect to see an improvement in your health and wellbeing within two weeks of starting the programme. You might find that health problems you have been tolerating for years simply disappear. The body has amazing powers of self-healing that spring into action whenever we provide it with the right conditions. Making healthy dietary changes can be just the jump-start your body needs to rebuild its health.

Following a dairy-free diet is very easy provided that you take a bit of time to plan and prepare. There shouldn't be any difficulty making this programme part of your everyday life and you should be able to continue with your usual activities. You won't be stuck for meal ideas as Chapter 18 contains a selection of healthy and delicious dairy-free recipes provided by Jane Sen. These include dairy-free versions of 'creamy' sauces and soups, a dairy-free pizza that has a cheese-like texture, and a selection of mouth-watering desserts.

While food provides the nutrients we need to keep us healthy, it also is one of life's great pleasures. As you'll see for yourself when you experiment with the recipes and follow the eating plan, food can – and should be – both nutritious and delicious. So don't feel that you need to deprive yourself or follow a bland, tasteless diet in order to improve your health. Nothing could be further from the truth!

are dairy products healthy?

Cow's milk is an excellent food for baby cows. Whether it is healthy for humans is the subject of a huge and on-going debate. Dairy products contain calcium, certain B-vitamins and are a source of dietary protein. However, you certainly don't need to eat dairy in order to get these nutrients, as they are available in a number of other foods. Dairy products are often high in unhealthy saturated fat, and most cheese contains salt, moulds and a whole range of different additives. All dairy foods contain a type of fat that is pro-inflammatory, or 'mucus-forming'. It may also be the case that dairy is associated with a few serious health conditions, such as prostate cancer.

The friendly bacteria found in live yoghurt, however, has many health benefits. Although live yoghurt is much easier to digest than other dairy foods, non-dairy yoghurts are widely available, providing an alternative source of these healthy bacteria.

Arguments as to whether dairy products are healthy or unhealthy are to a certain extent irrelevant. What is relevant is each person's individual relationship to a specific food. So, rather than labelling a particular food 'good' or 'bad', a better approach is to ask 'is this food good or bad *for me?*' It is possible to develop an intolerance to absolutely any food. All health experts would agree that lettuce is healthy. But if you have developed an intolerance to lettuce, then it isn't healthy for you. Similarly, by following the steps in this book, you will find out whether or not dairy is a suitable food to include in your diet, irrespective of what different health experts may tell you.

While it is important to identify the food 'culprits' responsible for your symptoms, it is also helpful to consider what is going on within the body that might be causing it to react against a specific food. Food intolerance can occur for a number of reasons. Factors such as excessive stress or frequently using antibiotics can create certain conditions within the body that increase the likelihood that food intolerance will develop. What this means is that avoiding a particular food is only part of the solution. For this reason, a main theme of this book is to show you steps you can take to strengthen the body so that there is less chance of it reacting negatively to food in the future. Once these steps are taken, people often find they can reintroduce moderate amounts of an intolerant food into their diet. This process usually takes about three to four months. Whether or not you decide to include dairy in your diet after this period is a matter of personal choice.

dairy foods in our diet

About nine thousand years ago, there was a great shift in human society. We moved from being hunter-gatherers to creating agricultural communities. It was at this time that we began to domesticate animals and to drink animal milk. We started to make cheese about three thousand years later. Not all societies adopted the habit of drinking animal milk and eating cheese. Instead, the practice of using animal milks (from goats and sheep as well as cows) was confined to communities located in colder parts of the world, such as Northern Europe.

No living creatures, apart from humans, continue to drink milk in adulthood. And there are no creatures, apart from us, who

consume milk derived from another species. In evolutionary terms, nine thousand years is a very short period of time and there is evidence to suggest that our digestive system has not fully adapted to the addition of cow's milk in the diet. Cow's milk is substantially different from human milk, both at the molecular level and in terms of the nutrients it contains. A cow weighs about 1,600 lb, and the baby calf grows incredibly quickly. Cow's milk, which is absolutely perfect for baby cows, is designed to help this quick growth. Furthermore, a cow has not one but four stomachs, which suggests that its digestive system functions quite differently from ours.

Nowadays, most dairy foods are consumed in North America and Europe. In China, Japan, Southeast Asia, India, the Middle East and Africa – about three quarters of the world's population – dairy foods are only eaten infrequently, if at all. The amount of dairy foods found in the standard Western diet is much greater than previous generations. Our forefathers, even 50 years ago, did not have access to the extensive selection of cheeses, yoghurts and other dairy products we now find on our supermarket shelves. It's not uncommon for people eating a typical Western diet to consume dairy at every meal. We have milk on our cereal for breakfast, a cheese sandwich for lunch, a cream cake as an afternoon snack and yet more dairy with dinner (pizza, pasta sauces, creamy sauces with meat and the like). The fashion for designer coffees and other drinks such as tea, hot chocolate and milkshakes are another major source of dairy. Dairy products are also regularly used in all manner of processed foods such as cookies, soups, puddings and chocolate. These two factors – that our digestive system may not have fully adapted to cow's milk products, and the large amount of dairy we consume in our diets – are reasons why we may be susceptible to developing dairy intolerance.

are you intolerant to dairy?

Before going any further, it will be useful for you to spend a couple of minutes completing the following questionnaire. This will help you find out if you have a dairy intolerance. Simply answer yes or no to the following questions then add up your total score of 'yes' answers.

1. I suffer with constipation and/or diarrhoea   yes/no
2. I often experience abdominal bloating   yes/no
3. I often experience gas and flatulence   yes/no
4. I can get indigestion or a burning sensation in
    my stomach after eating dairy   yes/no
5. I can feel nauseous after consuming dairy foods   yes/no
6. I have an inflammatory bowel condition   yes/no
7. I've noticed that my energy levels can slump after
    eating dairy   yes/no
8. I regularly have a blocked and stuffy nose   yes/no
9. I often have a chesty cough or 'mucus' on my chest yes/no
10. I get joint aches and pains   yes/no
11. I crave milk, cheese and other foods containing dairy yes/no
12. My skin has a tendency to be spotty or dry   yes/no
13. I suffer with eczema and/or psoriasis   yes/no
14. I suffer with asthma   yes/no
15. I suffer with headaches or migraines   yes/no
16. I suffer with premenstrual syndrome   yes/no
17. I have a tendency towards depression   yes/no
18. I often feel tired even though I've had plenty of sleep yes/no
19. My energy levels can go up and down during the day yes/no
20. I often have fluid retention   yes/no
21. My weight can fluctuate up and down by a few
    pounds for no apparent reason   yes/no
22. I'm finding it hard to shed excess weight even
    though I make sure I watch what I eat   yes/no

The higher your score on this test, the more likely it is that you have an intolerance to dairy. However, even if you have just two or three symptoms, you may still benefit from the Dairy-free Detox Diet. This questionnaire cannot provide conclusive 'proof' that you are or are not dairy intolerant; it is designed to be a useful indicator. You will get a clearer understanding of the relationship between dairy and your health when you do the first stage of the diet.

It is important to have a chat with your doctor before you start the programme. Although your symptoms may be related to dairy intolerance,
they could equally be associated with other health problems. So it is
worth ruling out any other health conditions before you start.

Now that you have some indication as to whether or not dairy is associated with your health symptoms, let's move on and look at the reasons why
dairy is often implicated as a food intolerance culprit.

2: lactose intolerance

In one of her funniest movies, Meg Ryan is travelling by train through France to catch up with her boyfriend who's with another woman. She's met a Frenchman who is helping her in her pursuit (naturally, she later falls passionately in love with him). She's happily chatting away to the Frenchman (Kevin Kline) while indulging in several different types of French cheese. In the next scene her happy mood has turned to anguish as she yells 'lactose intolerance!' and rushes to the loo. This scene is designed to make us laugh but in real life lactose intolerance is anything but funny. It can cause immense distress and pain.

In my previous career in corporate banking, my boss was lactose intolerant. He had discovered his condition during a weekend relaxing alone at home where he was drinking lots of milk and eating cheese. He essentially 'overdosed' on dairy and had to be rushed to hospital with severe digestive pain, diarrhoea and vomiting. He hasn't touched dairy products since.

what is lactose intolerance?

Lactose is the carbohydrate (sugar) found in cow's milk and other dairy products. It is found in all types of milk, including human breast milk. To digest lactose properly, the small intestine produces an enzyme called lactase. When enough lactase is produced, the lactose in milk and dairy foods is converted into glucose and galactose, which the body then uses as energy. Lactose intolerance is a condition where very little or no lactase is made by the body. This means that the lactose in dairy foods passes through the digestive tract in an undigested state, where it ferments in the colon causing pain and discomfort.

When we are babies, we make lots of lactase so that we can properly digest the milk provided by our mother. But from the age of two onwards, the amount of this enzyme we make slowly but surely starts to decline. By the time we reach adulthood, many of us produce very small amounts of lactase. Throughout human history, until we started to drink animal milk, there was absolutely no need for the lactase enzyme after weaning. This is why lactose intolerance is extremely common. Scientists have now discovered that our ability to make lactase is determined by our genes. For more about this subject, see Chapter 16.

Some health experts suggest that a way to overcome lactose intolerance is to eat small portions of dairy regularly and to increase the amount gradually. This, it is believed, will stimulate the body to produce more lactase so that the problem eventually disappears. But if lactase production is controlled by our genes and it has taken nine thousand years for just a small percentage of people to develop the gene sequence to produce lactase in adulthood, this approach is unlikely to work.

The most common form of lactose intolerance, *primary lactose intolerance*, is due to this gradual decline of lactase from early childhood. A very small number of people are born without the ability to make lactase (*congenital lactose intolerance*), which means they are unable to tolerate any milk, including human breast milk. It is also possible to stop making lactase after a gastrointestinal problem, such as mild food poisoning, or after taking certain medications. This *secondary lactose intolerance* is usually temporary, which means that milk and dairy foods can be reintroduced into the diet at a later date.

what are the symptoms?

Lactose intolerance symptoms usually occur within 30 minutes to two hours after eating dairy products. The effects are severe and include:

- nausea
- bloating
- diarrhoea
- abdominal cramps
- wind

Prior to my boss's trip to the accident and emergency department, he had regularly consumed dairy foods without noticing symptoms. What happened during that particular weekend was that he had really gone to town on dairy by drinking lots of milk and snacking on cheese and pizza. In his particular case, the amount of dairy he could tolerate before he experienced any adverse symptoms was quite large. For other people, just a small mouthful of cheese can provoke a similar response. And for ultra-sensitive individuals, even the tiniest amount of lactose found in many prescription medicines can elicit a severe reaction.

Therefore, **the amount of lactose that will provoke severe digestive problems varies from person to person according to the amount of lactase each individual can produce. One glass of milk might be tolerated without a severe reaction whereas two glasses might result in violent diarrhoea.** However, this one glass of milk might still be associated with less severe symptoms such as abdominal bloating, indigestion and flatulence. This suggests that the lactose is still not being fully digested by the body, a condition usually referred to as *lactose maldigestion*. Because these symptoms aren't as extreme, the connection between eating dairy and these digestive problems might be overlooked. Furthermore, regularly eating lactose-containing foods when the body is unable to digest them properly can irritate the digestive system and increase the possibility of full-blown food intolerance problems developing.

Did You Know?

The lactose content of dairy foods varies considerably. In general, the higher the fat content, the lower the level of lactose. Thus milk has more lactose than either cream or butter. Certain cheeses, especially aged cheese, contain only residual amounts of lactose. Many people can often tolerate live yoghurt, even if they have a lactase deficiency, as even though lactose is still present, it has effectively been pre-digested by the friendly bacteria.

Using lactase supplements can help lactose intolerance or lactose maldigestion. These are available in tablet form, and taken before eating dairy foods. Milk that has been treated with lactase is also widely available from supermarkets. However, a deficiency of lactase is only one way in which dairy foods can provoke health symptoms, so lactase supplements are not necessarily the solution. Let's now have a look at how another component of dairy foods can provoke intolerance problems.

3: intolerance to dairy protein

Lactose intolerance (*see Chapter 2*) can set the stage for other problems with milk and dairy foods. The undigested lactose can irritate the digestive system, making it difficult for dairy foods to be tolerated by the body. The symptoms associated with dairy intolerance are much more diverse than those related to lactose intolerance. As well as digestive problems, dairy intolerance is linked to all manner of seemingly unrelated symptoms such as:

- respiratory problems
- fluid retention
- urticaria (hives)
- lack of energy
- premenstrual syndrome
- emotional fluctuations
- inability to concentrate
- headaches and migraines

Although these symptoms may seem unrelated, they generally have one common root cause – the triggering of an inflammatory response in the body.

Did You Know?

The good news is that dairy intolerance can, in many cases, be resolved by avoiding the food for a period of time while taking steps to strengthen the underlying physical systems involved. This means that, in the long term, most dairy intolerant people should be able to include modest amounts of dairy in their diets without experiencing adverse reactions, should they wish to do so.

When Robert suffers with a blocked nose and chest problems after eating an ice cream, he is experiencing symptoms associated with a dairy intolerance. **The symptoms are provoked by an immune reaction to casein, the protein component of dairy foods.** Casein is broken down by the digestive system into peptides (groups of amino acids). It's usually the case that people with dairy intolerance are not digesting casein adequately. When these peptides are not properly digested, they can irritate the lining of the gut wall. This, in turn, can make the walls of the gut more porous or 'leaky', allowing the partially digested proteins to seep through into the blood and body fluids. The body's immune system is primed to react to such unwelcome visitors. In the gut, this increases inflammation and changes the balance of digestive flora, provoking digestive problems such as bloating, wind and discomfort.

Our immune system is extremely sophisticated. We are constantly exposed to viruses and bacteria from the environment. Most of the time we don't get sick because our immune system is able to protect us from these potential invaders. Food intolerance is a situation where the immune system is responding in an inappropriate fashion. It no longer sees the offending food as harmless. Rather, it reacts to that food as if it were a foreign invader that needs to be destroyed. This immune reaction sparks off a range of responses such as the excess mucus that accumulates in Robert's respiratory system.

symptoms of dairy intolerance

headaches

When Judy came to see me about her frequent headaches, she had already made the connection between this problem and eating dairy foods. Whenever dairy products were a part of her diet, she would suffer with mild headaches three or four times a week. If she avoided all dairy foods, her headaches would disappear. Headaches and migraines are often associated with an immune response that provokes inflammation, in this instance a particular reaction that increases blood stickiness (cheese also contains certain protein compounds that can bring on a migraine in another way).

fluid retention

Fluid retention is extremely common in cases of food intolerance. Holding on to fluid within the cells is the body's way of protecting itself from what it perceives to be a harmful substance. Abdominal bloating is often related to fluid accumulating in the digestive tract in response to the presence of intolerant foods. Fluid can accumulate all over the body and is particularly stubborn to shift until the intolerant food is removed from the diet. This is just one of the many reasons why some people find losing weight extremely difficult when food intolerance is present. Even when a reduced-calorie diet is followed religiously, weight refuses to budge. The reason is that excess weight is in the form of fluid rather than fat.

tiredness

Food intolerance puts the body under a great deal of stress and strain. The immune system is working much harder than it needs to by dealing with what it perceives as foreign invaders (food molecules). In addition, increased gut leakiness allows toxins that should be eliminated from the body via the digestive tract to enter the body. This creates yet more work for the immune system, as well as the liver (whose job it is to deal with toxic substances) and the lymphatic system. This is one reason why food intolerance is often associated with tiredness and fatigue; a great deal of the body's energy – which could be used for other things such as going out and having fun – is being used up unnecessarily.

blood sugar problems

Food intolerance can also disrupt the way the body balances blood sugar levels. A blood sugar imbalance is associated with problems such as fatigue, lack of concentration, irritability and mood swings. Unstable blood sugar levels are also a major factor in premenstrual syndrome. When the intolerant food is removed from the diet, these conditions often stabilize naturally within a short period. A blood sugar imbalance also makes losing weight more difficult than it needs to be because the body will rapidly convert food into fatty tissue.

other symptoms

Eczema and psoriasis are conditions associated with excessive inflammation of the skin. An intolerant food can also irritate the lining of the digestive tract, promoting inflammation and provoking similar digestive symptoms to those found in lactose intolerance, such as bloating, flatulence, constipation or diarrhoea.

am I allergic or intolerant? what's the difference?

The immune system is involved with both food allergy and food intolerance, but the reactions that occur are somewhat different in each case.[1] **With a food allergy, the immune response is usually immediate. For example, someone with a nut allergy will have an instant, and potentially life-threatening, reaction as soon as he or she comes into contact with this food.** Symptoms include constriction in the throat, swelling and difficulty breathing. Sometimes collapse (anaphylactic shock) can occur which, if not treated immediately with medical support, can result in death.

The symptoms of a food intolerance, on the other hand, can occur any time up to 72 hours after eating the culprit food. Most of these immune reactions provoke an inflammatory response. This is most obvious when excess mucus clogs up the chest and nose. Swelling of the joints, accompanied by aches and pains, can also be a signal of too much inflammation within the body.

what causes food intolerance?

Many different factors can combine to bring about a food intolerance. Here we look at some of the most common causes. For further information on this subject, *see Chapter 16*.

an unhealthy gut

The digestive system is quite sensitive, so there are several ways in which the digestive tract can become leaky. A healthy individual has about 3 pounds of friendly bacteria residing in their gut. These bacteria have a number of vital roles to play in maintaining our health. In particular, they help to make sure that the gut wall remains strong. It is all too easy, however, to drastically reduce the levels of these friendly bacteria and run the risk of making the gut leaky. For example, taking antibiotics, anti-inflammatory medication, the contraceptive pill or steroid drugs will disrupt the healthy balance of our friendly bacteria. Stress also takes its toll. The type of diet we eat significantly affects the health of our friendly bacteria. A diet high in processed foods, caffeine, sugar and alcohol does not provide the right nutrients for these important bacteria to flourish.

a repetitive diet

Some scientists also believe that eating the same food day in, day out can somehow trigger the immune system into reacting unfavourably towards that food. This line of reasoning does make sense as the two most common culprits for food intolerance – dairy and wheat – are both frequently eaten in the typical Western diet. Importantly, both dairy and wheat are quite difficult foods for the body to digest.

children and food intolerance

The Dairy-free Detox Diet is intended for adults who may have a dairy intolerance problem. However, it is worth mentioning the relationship between children and dairy intolerance as it is a very common condition. Young children are particularly susceptible to developing either food intolerances or food allergies because their digestive systems are naturally very leaky. The leakiness of the gut is useful when we are very young because it allows antibodies and other important health-promoting substances found in human breast milk to be used to their full benefit. It's only from the age of three onwards that gut permeability is reduced. Breast-feeding your baby reduces the risk of him or her developing an allergy or intolerance to cow's milk by as much as 10 times. Avoiding cow's milk until the age of 12 months also reduces the likelihood of sensitivity to dairy developing.

The most common symptoms associated with a food allergy or intolerance in children are eczema, asthma and colic. Occasionally behavioural problems, such as attention deficit disorder, can also be provoked by food intolerance. As cow's milk and dairy products are very common culprits, you might like to have a dairy-free trial period of two weeks if your child is experiencing these problems. If these foods are implicated, you should expect to see some improvements in symptoms by the end of this period. Other foods to consider are wheat, eggs, soya products and peanuts. To determine whether or not these foods are involved, you can use the same approach of avoiding the particular food(s) for two weeks and assessing any improvements. Make sure you stock up on plenty of healthy alternatives, especially if you are avoiding a couple of foods. At the end of two weeks, reintroduce one food at a time and assess the reaction. Wait three days before you introduce the next food.

If dairy products are avoided for any length of time, it's very important that you make sure your child is getting adequate calcium and other nutrients. Provided a healthy diet is followed, getting adequate calcium really isn't that difficult (*see Chapter 13 and Appendix 4 for healthy non-dairy sources of calcium*). If your infant shows signs of food allergy (*see page 16*), especially if there is a family history of allergy, it is best to also avoid all nuts or seeds until at least 12 months of age. A nutritionist who specializes in working with children can help you develop a healthy diet for your child.

the depression connection

Colleen has been a friend since before I trained as a nutritionist. We were sitting by the seashore one day when she decided to tell me about a serious depression that had plagued her life several years previously. This depression was so bad that on many mornings she would wake up feeling suicidal. Her marriage eventually disintegrated and ended in divorce, something she feels was mainly attributable to her on-going low moods.

Colleen used to drink milk and eat dairy foods every day. Some time after her divorce, for no particular reason, she stopped eating dairy for a few days. To her amazement her depression lifted, but at this point she did not associate this change in her mood with cutting out dairy. After a short period, however, the connection between what she was eating and how she felt started to make sense to her. Eventually she decided to eliminate all dairy foods for two months to see what would happen. Once she did this, her mood lifted and she remained depression-free.

As a result, Colleen no longer eats dairy. Very occasionally, such as a special night out, she might have a small portion of food that contains dairy. But she knows that there will be a price to pay. The next day her old depressive symptoms will return with a vengeance and last for up to 48 hours. Colleen had no interest whatsoever in the topic of nutrition; she literally discovered the link between her mood and a particular food by 'accident'.

Depression is a highly complex illness that can be caused by a great number of factors. But there is plenty of evidence to suggest that diet may play a highly significant part in some cases. The main culprits in this respect are the protein molecules found in both dairy (casein) and wheat (gluten). When these partially-digested peptides seep through the gut wall into blood and body fluids they can, in susceptible people, affect the chemistry of the brain. Most people with food intolerance do not suffer with such an extreme depression as Colleen, but many people report that their mood does improve once the offending food is removed from the diet. Sensitivity to casein and/or gluten has been found to be a factor in some cases of schizophrenia.[2] Gluten- and casein-free diets may also offer some benefit to children suffering with autism. So far there is only a small amount of scientific evidence to support this approach but what there is certainly seems very encouraging.[3]

food cravings

People with food intolerance often have cravings for the very foods that make them ill. These cravings are thought to be caused by the effects on brain chemistry of proteins such as casein and gluten. By binding with certain brain receptors, these proteins appear to produce a 'feel-good' factor in the short-term. Dr Jonathan Brostoff, one of the UK's leading medical experts on food intolerance, suggests that a craving for the intolerant food occurs in about 50 per cent of cases of food intolerance.[4] Naturally, food cravings can seriously interfere with any type of weight-loss programme. These cravings are physical, rather than psychological, in nature, so they can be very difficult to overcome with willpower alone. When the culprit food is removed from the diet, these cravings subside, usually within a period of a few days. Chapter 12 outlines some other useful dietary strategies for dealing with cravings.

dairy fat

A food intolerance condition provokes an immune response that increases the amount of inflammation within the body. People with dairy intolerance get a double-whammy because dairy foods naturally encourage inflammation. As well as saturated fat, dairy foods contain a particular type of polyunsaturated fat called arachidonic acid, which triggers an inflammatory reaction in the body. It can therefore further provoke conditions such as migraines, joint pains, eczema and asthma. There are other types of dietary fat that help the body control inflammation by producing highly anti-inflammatory substances (*see Chapter 11*). However, a diet containing high amounts of arachidonic acid effectively blocks the ability of the body to use these anti-inflammatory fats. These same fats are involved with numerous other bodily functions, including maintaining hormone balance (a factor in premenstrual syndrome) and protecting the cardiovascular system.

In other words, if you have a dairy intolerance you are increasing your susceptibility to inflammatory conditions such as eczema via two alternative routes. The orthodox medical treatment for these types of condition is to prescribe anti-inflammatory drugs, which are often steroid-based medications or antibiotics. Although this can provide relief in the short-term, it doesn't offer a long-term solution. Furthermore, these types of drug stress the digestive system, increasing the likelihood that it will become excessively leaky. This can perpetuate the food intolerance cycle.

The good news is that there are lots of natural nutritional strategies that can help strengthen the digestive system and the other physical systems (such as the liver) involved in food intolerance. Getting the right balance of essential fats in the diet also helps the body control the amount of inflammation it is producing, which provides good support for all inflammatory conditions. You will learn about all of these approaches when you start the Dairy-free Detox Diet.

4: other relationships between dairy and health

Dairy foods can cause health problems other than intolerance, which we looked at in the last chapter. There is growing evidence of a link between dairy consumption and debilitating diseases such as heart disease, insulin-dependent diabetes and prostate cancer. Most people associate dairy foods with healthy bones. But, as you'll see later on in this chapter, there isn't any conclusive proof that this is the case. In fact, there are good reasons to believe that a high intake of dairy foods (in particular, high-protein cheeses) can actually deplete bone strength.

It's worth mentioning at the outset that the association found between dairy intake and heart disease, diabetes and prostate cancer is just that – an association. Although scientific studies always take account of known risk factors (such as smoking) when conducting their investigations, it is a big leap from finding a positive relationship between dairy intake and a particular disease to asserting that dairy *causes* the disease. More work needs to be done in these areas before anyone can make conclusive statements. In other words, scientific research does not claim that dairy causes heart disease (or diabetes or prostate cancer) but if you know that you have a higher risk of getting this disease, you may wish to bear these research findings in mind.

heart disease

The association between a diet high in saturated fat and developing heart disease is now widely accepted. The main sources of saturated fat in the diet are dairy foods (whole milk, butter and cheese), meat and eggs. Although fish contains modest amounts of saturated fat, it is balanced by lots of heart-healthy 'omega-3' fats. Over the last decade or so, there has been a general shift away from high-fat dairy foods in favour of the less fatty options, such as the switch from whole milk to skimmed milk.

However, research studies have found that a high intake of low-fat dairy products, including skimmed milk, is also associated with an increased risk of cardiovascular disease.[1] This suggests that there are other components of dairy products, aside from saturated fat, that may be contributing to this problem. For more on these components, *see Chapter 16.*

prostate cancer

Too much calcium in the diet may also be linked with prostate cancer, the most common form of cancer and the leading cause of cancer death among men. **There is now substantial evidence of a clear link between dairy consumption and prostate cancer risk. Countries where lots of dairy foods are consumed have a much higher rate of prostate cancer than countries in which low amounts of dairy are eaten.**

A recent study monitored the diet and lifestyle of 20,000 men for 11 years. After accounting for other risk factors such as smoking, men who consumed 600 mg or more of calcium from dairy foods each day had a 34 per cent increased risk of getting prostate cancer than those who ate low amounts of dairy. It was also found that each additional 500 mg of calcium per day from dairy products increased the risk of prostate cancer by 16 per cent.[2] The link between dairy and prostate cancer has been reported in many other scientific studies.[3]

One proposed reason for this link is the high calcium content of dairy foods. High levels of calcium cause hormonal changes that reduce the body's ability to protect the cells of the prostate gland. Calcium supplements or non-dairy foods that are high in calcium would also increase the risk in the same way.

Saturated fats found in dairy products, meat and eggs are also considered a risk factor for prostate cancer. Furthermore, the use of hormones in dairy farming may also increase the risk of this disease (*see Chapter 15*). To protect against prostate cancer, experts recommend a diet high in lycopene (an antioxidant found in watermelon and tomatoes), vitamin E, selenium and omega-3 fats (found in oily fish).

childhood diabetes

There is mounting evidence that a high intake of cow's milk and other dairy products in early childhood is associated with the development of insulin-dependent diabetes mellitus (type one diabetes) in children who have a genetic susceptibility to the disease.

Type one diabetes is a genetic disorder so it is not 'caused' by drinking cow's milk. But, researchers are suggesting that a particular part of the protein found in cow's milk and dairy products mimics a specific antigen that provokes the immune system to attack the cells of the pancreas.[4] Therefore, dairy products may act as trigger in the development of insulin-dependent diabetes in susceptible individuals.[5] The younger the child is when cow's milk is introduced into the diet, the greater the risk of this occurring.[6]

do dairy products protect bones?

The most common concern of people who, for whatever reason, are avoiding dairy products is 'how will I protect my bones?' **The message 'eat dairy foods to keep your bones strong' has been drummed into us like a mantra since childhood. Yet it is quite possible to maintain bone health without having dairy in the diet.** If this wasn't true, then the billions of people on this planet who have never eaten dairy would be having problems. Of course, this is not the case.

There has been a lot of research on the relationship between dairy consumption and bone health. While a few studies do show that dairy has a protective effect, there is certainly no conclusive evidence that eating dairy products will protect our bones. In fact, rates of osteoporosis (brittle bones) are higher in countries that consume lots of dairy foods than in those whose intake of these products is low.[7]

An interesting piece of research undertaken by scientists from Harvard Medical School monitored the eating habits of nearly 80,000 female nurses for a period of 12 years. At the end of this time, the women who ate lots of dairy foods had no greater bone density than women who rarely consumed dairy. However, it was also found that the women who drank two or more glasses of milk each day had a 45 per cent *greater* risk of experiencing a hip fracture than those who drank modest amounts of milk.[8]

Another group of Harvard researchers followed a group of 40,000 professional men for eight years. The incidence of fractures was not significantly different for those who consumed dairy compared with those who did not. The same was true for total calcium intake, whether from dairy, other food sources or supplements. Those consuming high amounts of calcium (more than 1227 mg) had the same incidence of fractures as those who consumed low calcium (less than 512 mg).[9] Similar findings have been reported elsewhere. Two scientists from the University of Alabama recently assessed the whole body of research on dairy foods and bone health and summed up their findings by stating 'the body of scientific evidence appears inadequate to support a recommendation for daily intake of dairy foods to promote bone health'.[10]

There are convincing arguments as to why dairy products may actually deplete rather than strengthen bones. The body uses calcium and other minerals during the process of metabolizing protein foods. Our bones act as a mineral bank account that the body can make withdrawals from whenever more mineral supplies are needed. For example, eating 100 grams of cottage cheese provides us with about 61 mg of calcium. Yet the body needs to use a whopping 360 mg of calcium in order to deal with the metabolic by-products generated from the cottage cheese.[11] The deficit of 299 mg needs to come from somewhere and, unless there are other dietary sources of calcium that it can use, the body will take this amount of calcium from bones. Thus, rather than improving bone density, the cottage cheese has actually depleted it. While cottage cheese is one of the worst offenders in this respect, many other high-protein cheeses have the same type of impact. The process that makes this happen is discussed in more depth in Chapter 5.

So, it's certainly not the case that simply eating dairy products will guarantee us strong bones for life. And there is also reason to believe that a high consumption of dairy, without due regard for other important dietary and lifestyle factors, may in fact be detrimental to bone health. What is clear is that we can definitely maintain bone health on a dairy-free diet. You can read more about what you can do to keep your bones strong and healthy in Chapter 14.

colon cancer

Although a high intake of calcium appears to increase the risk of prostate cancer and heart disease, it is associated with a reduced risk of colon cancer. A large amount of red meat in the diet can damage the digestive tract, increasing the risk of colon cancer. Calcium appears to offset the unhealthy reaction provoked by eating meat.[12] However, perhaps a better approach for protecting our digestive tract would be to reduce the amount of red meat we eat in favour of fish and vegetarian sources of protein, rather than increasing calcium intake.

Another type of fat found in dairy products and meat is conjugated linoleic acid (CLA). CLA has been found to have a protective effect against certain cancers in animals[13] but whether it has the same effect in humans is as yet unclear.

5: the benefits of going alkaline

We tend to think of food in terms of the three main groups – protein, carbohydrate and fat. But another useful way of classifying foods is in terms of acid–alkaline balance. You've probably noticed that your mood and energy levels can change quite significantly depending upon what you've just eaten. Some meals can leave us feeling sluggish, bloated, irritable and tense while others have an energizing and uplifting effect. Although there are other reasons why food can have this impact, the most important is whether the meal has had an acidifying or alkalizing effect on the body.

acid-forming foods

Acid-forming foods – such as cheese, meat and some grains – can drain us of energy or make us feel 'wired' and hyper. It's no surprise that most people fall asleep on the sofa after eating Christmas lunch, as the meal is mainly acid-forming. On the other hand, alkaline-forming foods, found in abundance in fruits and vegetables, have the opposite effect, making us feel full of energy, calm and positive.

alkaline-forming foods

On the Dairy-free Detox Diet, you are encouraged to eat lots of fruits and vegetables and to drink freshly-made vegetable juices. **Fruits, vegetables and vegetable juices are alkaline-forming foods. Increasing the amount of these foods in the diet can have tremendous**

health-boosting effects. An alkaline-forming diet is a real energy booster, which means we will need less sleep and can achieve more with our day. It can significantly improve our mood so that we feel happier and less prone to becoming stressed out by life's problems. I always make sure that I eat lots of alkaline-forming foods when I'm involved with a big project, such as writing this book, as it helps to keep my mind clear and sharp as well as sparking off some creative moments.

In addition, alkaline-forming foods have a protective effect on our overall health in the long-term, reducing our risk of osteoporosis and a whole host of other diseases. The reason for the differing effects of acid-forming and alkaline-forming foods is due to what happens at a cellular level after food has been eaten. To find out more about this, *see Chapter 16.*

why acid–alkaline balance is important

In general, high-protein foods such as cheese, meat and fish, and also grains such as wheat and oats, are acid-forming. Most fruits and vegetables are alkaline-forming. Fats, oils and sugar are neutral in this respect.

The natural, healthy state of the whole body (apart from the digestive tract) is alkaline. In fact, body fluids (such as the blood and lymph) are kept within a very strict alkaline range. As the health of cells depends on them being alkaline, the acid created after eating a meal such as eggs and bacon could, if left untreated, cause cellular damage. Therefore, the body has devised a clever strategy to make sure that this doesn't happen. For more about this, *see Chapter 16.*

the acid-forming effect of cheese

How different foods affect the body is shown below. Positive numbers indicate acid-forming foods whereas negative numbers indicate alkaline-forming foods. Fats and oils are neutral. Acid-forming foods can vary substantially in their effects upon the body. When it comes to dairy products, different effects are seen according to the type of food. Most hard cheeses, which contain lots of protein, are extremely acid-forming. Cream cheese, which contains far less protein, has a slightly lower acid-forming potential than meat.

When the diet fails to provide enough alkaline minerals – particularly sodium, calcium, magnesium and potassium – the body uses the supply found in the bones, which is mainly calcium. In other words, **eating a piece of hard cheese such as cheddar, rather than supplying calcium, can actually cause calcium (and other minerals) to be lost from the body.** Acid-curd cheese, such as cottage cheese, has the same type of effect. On the other hand, milk and yoghurt have only a very minimal impact on acid–alkaline balance while butter has zero effect. This process is one reason why many research studies have found that a diet containing lots of dairy products is not associated with greater bone mass and has actually been found to decrease bone mass. Therefore, if dairy products can be tolerated in the diet, it is wise to choose those that have a less acid-forming effect and to keep the intake of hard cheeses and cottage cheese to a minimum.

Acid Load of Various Foods[1]

	Potential Renal Acid Load per 100 grams
Cheese – higher protein*	+23.6
Meat and meat products	+9.5
Cheese – lower protein**	+8.0
Fish	+7.9
Wheat flour	+7.0
Spaghetti	+6.7
Other grain products	+3.5
Milk and yoghurt	+1.0
Fats and oils	0.0
Vegetables	–2.8
Fruit and fruit juices	–3.1

* Higher-protein cheeses are those containing more than 15 grams protein/100g, which includes most cheese such as cheddar, brie, stilton and gruyère.
** Lower-protein cheeses are those containing less than 15 grams protein/100g, principally cream cheese.

getting the balance right

As the body's natural state is alkaline, it is no wonder that eating a high acid-forming diet over the long term is going to take its toll on our health and wellbeing. Of course, a certain amount of acid-forming foods are necessary in the diet. All foods that contain protein are acid-forming, but we definitely need sufficient protein in our diet for essential functions such as:

- repairing damaged cells
- making hormones
- keeping the brain functioning at its best
- rebuilding damaged bone

Animal sources of protein, such as dairy and meat, have a greater acid-forming potential than vegetable sources such as soya and legumes.

What is important is the overall balance between acid and alkaline foods in the diet. A typical modern diet containing lots of processed foods and only a few fruits and vegetables may consist of as much as 80–90 per cent acid- to 10–20 per cent alkaline-forming foods. Eating such a diet day in, day out will make us:

- mentally groggy
- lack physical energy and vitality
- more likely to experience aches and pains
- more likely to succumb to serious diseases such as osteoporosis or heart disease

---

Did You Know?

The symptoms of a hangover – headache, lack of energy and mental fatigue – are the result of the body becoming overly acidic and dehydrated. Eating an acid-forming diet over the long term is equivalent to continually experiencing the effects of a hangover without having the fun of the night before!

stress

Stress is a major problem for many people, given the fast pace of life we all experience. An acid-forming diet makes us much more susceptible to stress because of its effect on our mood and outlook on life. If we are constantly feeling mentally groggy and emotionally hyper, the problems we encounter in our everyday life are likely to have a far greater impact. In other words, eating lots of acid-forming foods essentially means we are not as centred and balanced as we could be. And it's not just food that creates excess acidity. Every time we feel stressed we release a series of hormones into our bloodstream that also increases the level of acidity in our body, thereby perpetuating the cycle.

an ideal balance

Therefore, one of the simplest but most effective things we can do to improve our health and wellbeing is to tip the acid–alkaline balance of our diet in favour of alkaline-forming foods. An ideal balance is in the region of 70–80 per cent alkaline-forming to 20–30 per cent acid-forming. This is often completely the opposite of what many people are eating! A mainly alkaline-forming diet provides a good foundation for helping the body to overcome any type of food intolerance problem. Eating in this way frees a lot of physical energy that can be used to restore lost health and vitality. An alkaline-forming diet also helps the body to reduce inflammation, a factor in conditions such as eczema, asthma and migraines.

Furthermore, because alkaline-forming foods require a lot less work to be metabolized, eating this type of diet usually results in a big increase in energy levels. **Many people report that minor health complaints such as aches and pains, headaches and difficulty concentrating disappear completely within a few weeks of eating a more alkaline-forming diet. Our mood usually improves and we begin to experience more joy and happiness in our day-to-day life. And, in the long term, we are doing a lot to enhance our health by reducing the risk of osteoporosis and other serious diseases.** Alkaline-forming foods also help the body to shift any excess fluid, so that we look and feel better. An important bonus is that increasing our intake of alkaline-forming fruits and vegetables will also ensure we are getting a whole spectrum of antioxidant vitamins and minerals, fibre and other valuable nutrients. These all have fantastic health-promoting benefits in other ways.

Unless you have a complete aversion to all fruits and vegetables, tilting the scales in favour of alkaline-forming foods doesn't require a radical change of diet. There are lots of simple strategies that can help you get the right balance between these two food groups. Chapter 7, which outlines the foods to eat and avoid during the Dairy-free Detox Diet, has a few suggestions for easy ways of increasing your intake of alkaline-forming foods. You'll be pleasantly surprised at the positive effect such a simple strategy can have on your overall health.

6: the two-week programme

Amanda is a very attractive woman in her late 20s. She visited my clinic to find out whether changes to her diet might help her overcome troublesome skin problems. She had been suffering with dry and spotty skin for some time, which was interfering with her career as a photographic model. After analysing her eating habits and other health symptoms, I suggested she avoid all dairy foods for two weeks to see if this helped. When she came for her next appointment, the improvement in her skin was obvious. She also told me she had more energy and that her stomach was no longer bloated.

Inspired by her success, her husband Peter arranged to come and see me. He was experiencing lots of digestive problems as well as frequent headaches. Again, the dietary culprit appeared to be dairy products so he agreed to avoid these foods for two weeks. I also recommended certain foods and nutritional supplements that would support his digestive system. Peter responded very well to the two-week dairy avoidance. His digestive symptoms improved and his headaches disappeared completely. Amanda and Peter continued to avoid dairy for three months, while making sure they were eating a healthy, nutritious diet. At the end of this period, they both found that they remained symptom-free as long as they kept their dairy intake to a minimum.

what is the dairy-free detox diet?

For most people, avoiding a suspected intolerant food for a period of two weeks is plenty of time to determine whether or not this food is associated with any health symptoms. There are lots of food-intolerance tests on the market, but the easiest, cheapest and most accurate approach is usually to avoid eating the suspect food and monitor any changes to your well-being. This is what you will be doing during the first stage of the Dairy-free Detox Diet.

In addition to avoiding all sources of dairy, you will be taking some simple steps to strengthen the underlying body systems that are frequently involved with food intolerance. This is achieved by including specific foods that have a healing and strengthening effect on the body and by using a few key nutritional supplements. **The eating plan you will be following is a nutrient-rich, alkaline-forming diet that will support your overall health in many different ways. In addition, it will help you lose weight, should you need to, without all the fuss of calorie counting or the side-effects of dieting, such as feeling hungry all the time.**

A 'detox' generally refers to a way of 'spring-cleaning' the body, but this is not the purpose of the Dairy-free Detox Diet. Rather, this programme is solely concerned with helping you identify whether or not you have an intolerance to dairy foods and outlining the steps you can take to heal this condition. If you are interested in trying a detox of the spring-cleaning variety, have a look at my book *Super Energy Detox* (Thorsons). I find detoxing an extremely beneficial thing to do once or twice a year.

The Dairy-free Detox Diet is really easy to follow. But the key to making it work is a bit of preparation and planning, both beforehand and during the programme itself. This chapter discusses important issues, such as the changes you might expect to experience during these two weeks and how to prepare effectively. There is also a section on the different types of intolerance tests available, should you be interested in exploring these options.

what to expect

withdrawal symptoms

Some people, but by no means all, experience a few minor withdrawal symptoms when they remove an intolerant food from the diet. Withdrawal symptoms usually consist of things like:

- a mild headache
- feeling overly tired
- inability to concentrate
- feeling a bit 'spacey'

The digestive system might also react; it's not unusual to experience slight constipation and/or diarrhoea during the first few days. Sometimes people might experience a more severe reaction, such as flu-like symptoms and/or joint swelling. All of these withdrawal symptoms, if they happen at all, usually pass within a maximum of five or six days.

In fact, withdrawal symptoms, while certainly not pleasant, should be viewed as a really good sign because they indicate that changes are happening within the body. So if you do experience any unusual minor health symptoms during the first few days, this can be interpreted as the first sign that you do have a dairy intolerance. If you are intolerant to dairy then, after getting through this initial reaction, the remainder of the two-week period should result in an overall improvement in your wellbeing. If you feel out of sorts for longer than a few days then check with your doctor, as it may be that something else is causing your symptoms.

improved digestion

Different health symptoms take different amounts of time to respond to dietary changes. **Digestive complaints are usually the first area to improve when an intolerant food is removed. Therefore, you should expect to experience less indigestion, wind and bloating and the like after about one week of the programme.** You will probably experience more frequent bowel movements because the types of food you will be eating contain lots of healthy soluble fibre. People who live in traditional tribal communities that typically eat a high-fibre diet usually have two to three bowel movements per day. Colon cancer is extremely rare in these communities. Increasing your intake of fibre can also help to reduce cholesterol.

more energy

Energy levels usually improve quite quickly once an intolerant food is removed from the diet. Many people report that they no longer feel groggy when they wake up in the morning and that they seem to achieve more during the day. The mind can start to feel clearer and sharper. Depression, if it is associated with dairy intolerance, can also lift, as in the case of Colleen, whom you met in Chapter 3.

fluid loss

You might also find yourself going to the loo quite frequently as your body starts to remove any excess fluid associated with a dairy intolerance. As a result, stomach bloating can significantly reduce. Facial puffiness, again provoked by excess fluid, can also disappear. Fluid loss will also translate into weight loss. This can vary from person to person from a couple of pounds to up to 10 pounds by the end of the two weeks. Weight loss related to the removal of excess fluid is much faster than shedding excess fat. The healthiest way to lose excess fat is to do it slowly, at a rate of about two pounds per week (*Chapter 12 discusses the topic of weight loss in more depth*).

other benefits

Conditions such as a blocked nose and mild headaches should improve during the latter half of the two-week period. Skin conditions such as eczema generally take somewhat longer to respond to dietary changes but nevertheless you should notice some improvement, especially if you take a supplement of essential fats (discussed in the next chapter). Other symptoms, such as premenstrual syndrome, may take up to three months to improve significantly from the time of removing an intolerant food while simultaneously making healthy dietary changes.

These are the usual types of changes that people experience when an intolerant food is removed from the diet. However, everybody is different.

So let your body adjust at the speed that suits it best. Sometimes people don't notice any difference in their health symptoms until 10 days or so into the programme. But if dairy intolerance is present, you should expect to experience quite a few changes by the end of 14 days. If you are taking any prescribed medication, don't stop taking it without discussing this with your doctor first, even if you feel much better.

when to start

When to start is really up to you. Make sure you have a check-up with your doctor first to be sure that any symptoms you are experiencing are not related to any other health condition. As some people do get minor withdrawal symptoms, you might like to start on a Friday so that you have the whole weekend to relax should you experience a headache or feel a bit tired. It's also worthwhile checking your diary for social commitments that might make following the programme tricky, such as going to a wedding where you might be tempted to indulge in some wedding cake.

stocking up

Once you have decided on a specific day to start, you need to go on a shopping trip to stock up on various dairy-free substitutes you may require and the specific healing foods you will be eating during the programme. There are also a few nutritional supplements to buy. Everything you need is outlined in the next two chapters. It's a good idea to buy all these things before you start. It's also helpful to clean out the fridge and some kitchen cupboards. Check the labels of foods such as cookies, sauces, soups and the like. If they contain dairy, put them in a separate cupboard. This way you won't inadvertently eat some dairy-containing foods. Likewise, you can create different sections in the fridge; a dairy section for other members of your family and a dairy-free section for you.

┌─ Tell Your Friends ────────────────────────────

It's helpful to let people know what you are doing so you don't end up in awkward situations. For example, if you are invited to a dinner party, pick up the phone and let your hosts know in advance that you are avoiding dairy so they can make any necessary adjustments to the menu. This saves embarrassment later.

└──

monitoring your changes

The aim of this stage of the Dairy-free Detox Diet is for you to get a very clear idea as to whether or not dairy foods are involved in any of your health symptoms. Depending upon the improvements you experience, you may then decide to avoid dairy for a slightly longer period of time, usually at least three months. Everything you need to do on stage two of the programme is explained in Chapter 10.

When it comes to observing health changes, we all seem to suffer with a form of selective memory. I've noticed this in myself and in people who come to me for nutritional support. This is particularly true for less important health problems. Once a minor symptom has cleared up, we seem to forget that we ever used to suffer with this condition! For example, I might ask someone how a particular health problem has changed since the last time we met. Often this will be met with a puzzled expression. I then remind her that the last time she was at the clinic she said she suffered with this problem most of the time. 'Oh that! Well, I haven't had that now for at least four weeks' is the usual response. Of course, the only reason I remember these different symptoms is because I keep very detailed client records.

To overcome this tendency to have a selective memory, it is really helpful to keep a record of all your health symptoms both before and after stage one of the Dairy-free Detox Diet. This will give you a really accurate assessment of the relationship between dairy and your health.

So before you start the programme, take a few minutes to complete the following assessment. This assessment contains many of the symptoms that can be associated with dairy intolerance, or food intolerance in general, but of course they could relate to other nutritional conditions such as vitamin deficiencies. Premenstrual syndrome, which can be exacerbated by food intolerance, has not been included on the assessment as two weeks is insufficient time to notice a significant improvement.

There is space for you to include any additional personal symptoms that you believe might be associated with a dairy intolerance. A similar assessment is provided in Chapter 10, which you should complete after you have finished the two-week programme.

Pre-detox Assessment

	None	Mild	Moderate	Severe
Indigestion				
Flatulence				
Constipation				
Diarrhoea				
Abdominal bloating				
Blocked nose				
Chest congestion				
Eczema				
Asthma				
Poor skin				
Headaches				
Migraines				
Fluid retention				
Weight fluctuations				
Joint aches and pains				
Lack of energy				
Tiredness upon waking				
Depression				
Low mood				
Inability to concentrate				
Forgetfulness				
Other:				

a food and symptom diary

Here's something you might like to try if you feel so inclined and have sufficient time. During this two-week period, keep a daily record of everything you eat and drink. It's useful to carry a small notebook with you so you can write things down straightaway. Then, at the end of each day, you can also write a couple of sentences that sum up how you have been feeling. Short sentences such as 'I felt quite tired', 'I had loads of energy today', 'I had a mild headache' or 'my stomach bloating has gone' are all that you need.

These notes will give you really clear information about your health and wellbeing during the first stage of the programme. The food and symptom diary will also help you identify any other food intolerance problems you might be experiencing. Then, if you notice only a modest improvement by the end of this first stage of the programme, there is a written record to help you determine which other food(s) might also be involved.

testing for dairy intolerance

As mentioned, the simplest method for determining whether or not you have dairy intolerance is to eliminate this food for two weeks and monitor any changes. However, you might also be interested exploring the various testing options available, so I've outlined how some of these tests work. Information on laboratories that offer these tests is provided in Appendix 5, Useful Information and Addresses.

hydrogen breath test

This test is to find out whether or not someone has lactose intolerance (*see Chapter 2*). The test consists of drinking a liquid that contains some lactose and then testing to see if there is any hydrogen in the breath. When lactose is not digested properly, certain bacteria residing in the digestive tract cause it to ferment. This produces hydrogen gas, which is absorbed through the gut into the bloodstream and subsequently exhaled from the lungs. The test is not totally reliable and can also be disrupted by factors such as smoking and certain drugs. It is not usually used with young children. Your doctor can arrange for you to take the test.

ELISA test

ELISA stands for 'enzyme-linked immunosorbent assay' and is useful for assessing dairy intolerance and intolerance to any other food. Blood is tested for IgG antibodies (the immune response associated with intolerance) against particular foods. A raised level of IgG antibodies against, say, dairy foods would provide strong evidence that there is intolerance to dairy. The test usually assesses antibodies against 50 to 100 different foods. It is done via the post, which makes it very easy. Only a drop or two of blood is needed, which you take yourself using the pin-prick device in the kit. You then post this to the laboratory, which will provide your test results within a week or two. The ELISA test is not normally available from your doctor so you will need to pay for it privately. Many private health-care policies will meet the cost of this test, so contact your provider and check. A nutritionist can help to organize this for you, or you can do it yourself. Although it can be somewhat expensive, it is quite reliable.

rast test

This stands for 'radioallergosorbent' test and is useful for finding out whether there is an allergy to a particular food. It measures the presence of IgE antibodies (the immune response associated with an allergy) in the blood against different types of foods. The Rast test can sometimes provide inaccurate results. It can be a useful complement to the ELISA test to determine whether a reaction to dairy is provoked by either an intolerance or an allergy. Your doctor should be able to arrange a Rast test for you.

gut permeability test

This test assesses whether the digestive tract has become too leaky. You collect a urine sample after drinking a small amount of liquid that contains specific neutral carbohydrate molecules. When the gut is too leaky, a large proportion of these molecules will seep through the gut wall into body fluids. These molecules are subsequently eliminated in the urine. Therefore the amount of molecules in the urine determines whether or not the gut has become too leaky. A postal service for this test is available. You need your doctor's consent but you will probably have to pay for it from your own funds. Part of the nutritional protocol for dealing with a food intolerance condition is to improve the health of the digestive system, so this test can provide useful information.

urine peptide test

Although not frequently used, this test can be very useful in certain circumstances. The purpose of the test is to see whether there are casein peptides in the urine. Casein peptides can only appear in the urine if these proteins have not been digested properly. As with the gut permeability test, the partially-digested peptides seep through the gut wall into body fluids and will then be eliminated in urine. This test might be useful for people suffering with depression or mood disorders. As for the gut permeability test, you collect a sample of your urine and send it to the laboratory.

7: foods to eat

Following a dairy-free diet is really very easy and should not cause any major problems in your day-to-day life. This chapter outlines all of the foods you need to avoid or cut down on while following the two-week Dairy-free Detox programme. You will also learn about the types of food to include in your diet. You'll find a few tips about eating out and what to do if you are away from home. All in all, you should sail through the next couple of weeks without any problems.

The eating guidelines you will read about here are pretty much the same as those you will follow during stage two of the programme. In fact, these dietary principles provide an excellent foundation for developing a healthy-eating plan in the longer term. Topics you'll read about later, such as the importance of essential fats, will give you more information about healthy eating after you've completed the programme.

avoiding dairy

Look upon the next two weeks as a scientific experiment you are conducting on yourself. In order to get a clear result, it is very important that you make sure you avoid all sources of dairy throughout this period. Sometimes people get a bit confused about exactly what foods belong to the dairy family. Here, the term dairy relates to any product that comes from cow's milk, namely:

- milk
- cream

- yoghurt
- fromage frais
- cheese
- butter

processed foods

Dairy products are also widely used in many processed foods. These include foods like:

- quiche
- pizza
- cakes
- chocolate
- soups
- sauces
- instant hot drinks such as Ovaltine

If you have most of your meals at home, you are more in control of what you are eating, either by making meals from scratch or by checking the ingredients labels of any prepared products you purchase. If you eat away from home a lot, it is worth checking ingredients if in doubt. Some tips for eating out are given below. Have a look at Appendix 2 for a list of foods that contain dairy and for terms used on labels (such as whey or caseinates) that indicate dairy is present in the product.

If you do have some dairy by mistake, don't worry. Just resume the dairy-free plan the next day. It's worth noting that if this happens during the later stages of the two weeks, you might experience a reaction. After avoiding an intolerant food for even a week or so, the body can become highly sensitized to this food. This increased sensitivity may provoke a reaction, such as suddenly feeling hot and sweaty, or a recurrence of symptoms that have cleared up. This reaction will usually pass within a few hours.

avoiding other milk-based products

Milk, yoghurt and cheese from other animals, such as goats and sheep, can sometimes be tolerated by people who have an intolerance to dairy foods. However, during this first phase of the Dairy-free Detox Diet, it is best if you avoid all these foods. Goat's and sheep's milk products also contain lactose and casein, although in a slightly different form to that found in cow's milk foods. Therefore, in order to get a really accurate indication of the relationship between dairy and your health, you need to avoid these foods as well for the time being. You may be able to include these foods in stage two of the programme.

dairy substitutes

Nowadays there are plenty of dairy-free milk substitutes available. These include soya milk, rice milk and oat milk. You can get all of these from the larger supermarkets. The dairy-free milks are very useful for breakfast cereals and in cooking. Individual tastes do vary so not everyone likes them. I really like rice milk and always use it on breakfast cereals such as porridge or buckwheat. In the winter I heat up some rice milk and add half a teaspoon of organic cocoa powder, which makes an excellent dairy-free hot chocolate. Rice milk is not suitable for tea and coffee, but you can try soya milk. The flavour of soya milk varies considerably from brand to brand so try a couple of different products to see which suits you best. Soya cream is also widely available and makes a good substitute for single cream.

soya foods

Soya foods are healthy foods to include in your diet. They help to balance hormones so can be beneficial for women suffering from premenstrual syndrome or menopausal symptoms. They may also help keep your bones healthy.[1] Soya foods are also a good source of dietary protein. Tofu is a versatile and healthy food. If you haven't cooked with tofu before, have a look at Jane's recipes in Chapter 18 for a few tasty ideas.

Dairy-free milk substitutes aren't compulsory, as you can easily manage without them. For example, breakfast cereals such as muesli taste quite good with a combination of apple juice and water. Cutting back on tea and coffee in favour of herb teas will reduce your need for substitute milks. Reducing caffeine is better for your health as well.

Soya yoghurt can make a healthy addition to a dairy-free diet as it contains 'friendly' bacteria (*see page 65, below*). It is available, either plain or with fruit, from most supermarkets. The plain version goes well with a fresh fruit salad. Soya desserts, which are also readily available at supermarkets, make a healthy and delicious alternative to custard. You can buy soya ice cream (read the label to make sure it doesn't contain hydrogenated fat), or alternatively you could have fruit sorbet.

Good News for Chocoholics

Most chocolate contains dairy but there are some dairy-free versions so there is no reason to feel deprived. Look out for Green and Black's organic dark chocolate, which is dairy-free. One small piece will satisfy any chocolate craving you might have. However, if you suffer with headaches or migraines, it's best to avoid chocolate.

dairy-free processed foods

Nowadays there are lots of processed foods targeted at people who don't eat dairy. These include products like dairy-free cheese, which is usually made from soya. However, if the product is highly processed, it is not really that good for your health so use your discretion when shopping. Also note that **if the label just says 'lactose-free' then it will still contain either dairy casein and/or dairy fat. Lactose-free rice 'cheese' contains casein, so avoid this product.** All the terms you need to look out for on labels are provided in Appendix 2. Creating healthy menus that don't require dairy is really quite easy. Jane has provided you with plenty of healthy and delicious dairy-free recipes in Chapter 18, so you shouldn't be stuck for ideas.

foods to eat

The foods you are encouraged to eat on this programme have all been selected because they are rich in nutrients and provide lots of benefits for your health and wellbeing. A healthy diet should contain a good balance of protein, carbohydrate and essential fats. Protein is needed for many functions, such as repairing damaged cells and making hormones. Carbohydrates are our main source of energy. Essential fats are involved in virtually every body system, including the healthy functioning of the brain, nervous system, hormones and skin.

You need to make sure you are getting a proper balance of these three food groups. More importantly, you need to make sure you are choosing healthy options from each group.

carbohydrates

Carbohydrate foods vary considerably in terms of both nutrient content and the effect they have on our health. Sugar is a carbohydrate but it contains virtually no nutrients. A high-sugar diet can lead to blood sugar imbalances, diabetes, heart disease and weight gain. In contrast, porridge is also a carbohydrate but it is a valuable source of B-vitamins and helps to stabilize, rather than disrupt, blood-sugar balance. Porridge is also high in soluble fibre, which helps keep our digestive system healthy.

Complex carbohydrates are the ones to go for as they usually release their energy slowly and provide plenty of nutrients and fibre. The chart below provides a selection for you to try. There is more information on carbohydrates in Chapter 12, which discusses how to overcome cravings for good and achieve healthy and permanent weight loss.

protein

Vegetarian sources of protein are generally healthier than animal sources. They are less acid-forming and do not contain the unhealthy saturated fats found in meat. Many vegetarian sources of protein also contain good quality carbohydrates. Cooking rice and lentils together, both of which are usually considered carbohydrate foods, will also provide you with a complete source of protein. You might like to try quinoa, which is an excellent source of protein and carbohydrate. You simply boil it in a little water for about 15 minutes. It is rather bland so can benefit from some herbs and spices.

Other good sources of protein are chickpeas (houmous), beans and tofu. Fish is another excellent protein source and it also contains plenty of omega-3 fats, which have lots of health-promoting benefits, including protecting your heart. If you eat meat, then fresh lean meats, preferably organic, are far better than processed meats (which should be avoided as they contain lots of additives).

Did You Know?

Although protein is important, we don't need that much of it to keep healthy. Most of us could benefit from cutting back on our protein intake. On average, men consume 85 grams per day, which is more than 50 per cent above the UK government recommendation of 55.5 grams. Women consume an average of 62 grams, far above the recommended 45 grams. You should be able to meet all your needs with two-to-three moderate-sized servings of protein foods per day. As always, quality is better than quantity.

essential fats

One serving of essential fats, which amounts to a handful of seeds and nuts or one tablespoon of oil, is sufficient to meet our daily requirements. If you eat fish, try to have oily fish such as salmon a few times each week for its omega-3 fats, which are useful in food-intolerance conditions (there's more on essential fats in Chapter 11).

a healthy balance

You should aim to have three meals per day and a couple of healthy snacks if you feel peckish. This also applies if you are trying to lose weight. Eating regular meals will help keep your energy levels buoyant and blood sugar balanced. You'll find some healthy food choices in the table below.

Protein	Carbohydrate	Essential fats	Alkaline-forming
Quinoa	Brown rice	Flax seeds	Fresh fruit
Tofu & soya foods	Beans	Sesame seeds	Dried fruit
Lentils & legumes	Barley	Pumpkin seeds	Vegetables
Nuts	Chickpeas	Walnuts	Fruit juices
Seeds	Porridge	Oily fish	Vegetable juices
Fish	Lentils & legumes	Sunflower seeds	
Lean meat	Millet	Tahini	
Eggs	Corn	Vegetable oils	
Sea vegetables	Wholegrain bread		
2–3 servings	3–4 servings	1 serving	5–6+ servings

variety

Try to get as much variety into your diet as you can. It's useful to rotate the foods you eat so you don't eat the same foods every day. From the carbohydrate category, for example, you could choose brown rice one day, baked potatoes the next and beans the day after that. This will help ensure that you get the full spectrum of vitamins and minerals you need to keep healthy.

going alkaline

Jessica is a mother of two who also works full time as an accountant. She came to see me about her digestive problems, premenstrual syndrome and lack of energy. She also said that she felt overwhelmed, irritable and mildly depressed a lot of the time and that life seemed to have been reduced to one long struggle. A typical diet for Jessica consisted of cereal for breakfast, some type of sandwich for lunch and ready meals for dinner. Although she made sure there was always plenty of fruit and vegetables available for her children, she rarely ate these foods herself. Her total fluid intake consisted of coffee and tea during the day and a couple of glasses of wine in the evening.

Once I explained to Jessica how the body's acid–alkaline balance could affect mood and energy levels, she was keen to see how a shift towards alkaline-forming foods would impact on her overall wellbeing. She said she didn't feel she could sit down and munch on a big bowl of salad every day so I suggested a few simple strategies for increasing alkaline-forming foods. These included fresh vegetable juices, fruit smoothies and easy-to-prepare vegetable meals such as soups and stews.

When she returned to the clinic six weeks later, she reported that she had experienced a tremendous change in her health and mood. She was no longer snappy with colleagues and felt much more positive about life. She had lots of energy and, because her mind was clearer, she handled her workload with much less stress. As a committed convert to the value of an alkaline-forming diet, she said she would continue with her new way of eating in the long term.

Tipping the scales in favour of alkaline-forming foods is a good foundation for helping to heal a food-intolerance condition. Furthermore, a mainly alkaline-forming diet will help the body rid itself of excess fluid.

Aside from the substantial benefits to our mood and energy levels, alkaline-forming foods also contain valuable nutrients that support our health in many other ways. They are packed with antioxidant nutrients that reduce our risk of suffering from serious illnesses such as cancer or heart disease. They keep us looking younger for longer. And they contain plenty of soluble fibre, which is important for keeping our digestive system healthy. Here are some guidelines for making sure your diet contains enough alkaline-forming foods during the Dairy-free Detox Diet:

- Have at least two pieces of fresh fruit each day.
- Have a large portion of vegetables with lunch and dinner.
- Have one glass of freshly-prepared vegetable juice each day (*see the next chapter for information on vegetable juices*).
- Have one glass of freshly-squeezed fruit juice or a fruit smoothie every day.
- If you fancy something sweet, opt for dried fruits, such as apricots, raisins or sultanas.

Here are a few suggestions for other ways to increase your intake of alkaline-forming foods:

- Make vegetable-rich meals for your family such as chunky soups, stews and stir-fries. In the summer, make large mixed salads that contain a portion of protein, such as grilled chicken or tuna. Even the kids won't notice that their vegetable intake is increasing!
- Instead of crisps (chips), cookies or popcorn, have a plate of crudités with a tasty dip to nibble on for snacks.
- When fruits are plentiful during the summer, keep a freshly-made fruit salad in the fridge. It makes a convenient snack for all the family whenever anyone feels peckish.
- Whiz up some soft fruits in a blender with a little water to make a tasty fruit smoothie. The most die-hard fruit phobic usually succumbs to and enjoys a smoothie. This is also a great way of getting more fruit into children's diets.

- Choose the less acid-forming foods in favour of the higher ones. For example, cutting back on pasta and substituting rice would lower the overall acidity of your diet. It's also healthy to reduce red meat in favour of less acid-forming fish and vegetarian sources of protein.

getting enough calcium

Many people worry that they will not get enough calcium if they avoid dairy foods. But this need not be the case. The eating plan you will be following will provide you with lots of calcium-rich foods. Fish such as sardines, salmon and whitebait are excellent sources of calcium as are green leafy vegetables (excluding spinach, as the calcium is not absorbed properly). Calcium is also found in nuts and seeds, particularly almonds, sesame seeds and sunflower seeds. Nut butters such as almond and tahini (ground-up sesame seeds) provide a very good source of calcium and can be used on toast or as toppings. You can also purchase calcium-enriched tofu, soya milk and rice milk.

Calcium needs to be balanced with other minerals and vitamins if you are to get the full benefit of this nutrient. Dairy foods do not provide adequate amounts of these other nutrients, while the eating plan you will be following here does. As this is an important subject, I have devoted Chapter 13 to discussing it in some depth. Appendix 4 lists the calcium content of different foods.

foods to reduce

Although the main purpose of these two weeks is for you to assess whether or not dairy foods are the cause of your health symptoms, it will also be helpful for you to cut back on certain foods and drinks that do not particularly support your health. The foods either to avoid or keep to a minimum in your diet are:

- any products that are highly processed or refined
- foods that contain lots of sugar
- deep-fried food

caffeine and alcohol

Caffeine can disrupt blood sugar balance, perpetuate headaches and migraines and make us feel emotionally wired or stressed. So it's best to either avoid caffeine-containing drinks or to keep your intake low. Keep alcohol intake low as well.

wheat

Wheat is another common intolerant food. It can be hard on the digestive system so it's best not to overindulge in this food during these two weeks. There is no need to avoid it totally; just keep your intake moderate and rotate wheat with other grains.

salt

If you suffer with fluid retention, you would probably benefit from cutting down on salty foods and not adding salt to meals. Salt also reduces bone mass and contributes to high blood pressure so it is definitely not a healthy component of the diet. Many processed foods contain salt, so these are best avoided (such as crisps, bacon, processed meats and corn-flakes). Buy plain, unsalted nuts rather than those with added salt.

vegetable spreads

Don't use vegetable spreads as they contain harmful hydrogenated fats (also called trans fats). You can purchase unhydrogenated vegetable spreads at the health-food shop, but read the ingredients label to make sure it does not contain dairy (many vegetable spreads contain dairy). Alternatively, you can opt for nut butters or tahini, which will boost your calcium intake as well. The health problems associated with hydrogenated fats are discussed in Chapter 11.

water

It is important to drink at least 1.5 litres of water per day. This can be bottled mineral water or filtered tap water. **Drinking lots of water will help reduce your chances of experiencing withdrawal symptoms in the early stages of this two-week period.** Although it might sound paradoxical, drinking more water will actually help the body shift any excess fluid. This is because fluid retention is often a sign of dehydration within the body as well as a symptom associated with food intolerance.

It's a good idea to get into the habit of drinking lots of water each day in the longer term. The body loses about 1.5 litres of water per day; one third of this is exhaled from the lungs alone. If we want to be healthy, we need to replace this lost water. Being slightly dehydrated can reduce our energy levels, impair our mental functioning and make our skin look dull.

If you are not used to drinking this much water, it can be helpful to schedule in specific 'drinking times' during the day. You could 'programme' certain regular activities that happen during your day to act as reminders to have some water. Such activities could include every time you check the time, whenever you check your e-mails or any similar activity you do repeatedly. Don't drink too much water with meals as it dilutes the digestive enzymes, making the digestive system work harder than it needs to.

summary

Here is a summary of the main guidelines you need to follow during this stage of the Dairy-free Detox Diet:

Choose	Cut down	Avoid
2–3 servings of protein foods	Processed foods	Cow's milk
3–4 servings of carbohydrates	Sugary foods	Dairy yoghurt
1 serving of essential fats	Caffeine	Cheese
6 servings of fruit and vegetables	Alcohol	Butter
Vegetable and fruit juices	Wheat	Other foods with dairy
Nuts and seeds	Salt	Goat's milk products
Calcium-rich foods		Sheep's milk products
Dairy-free milk substitutes		Hydrogenated spreads
Soya foods		
Minimum of 1.5 litres water p/day		

Eat three meals a day plus snacks whenever you feel hungry.
Have plenty of variety.

cooking for the family

You should find it easy to fit your new eating plan into your usual activities, even if you are preparing food for your family. Breakfast and lunch are usually quick to prepare, so it shouldn't take much extra effort to make something different for yourself if the rest of your family is still eating dairy foods. There are literally hundreds of dairy-free choices for the evening meal, so you shouldn't need to concoct two different recipes. After all, the whole family will benefit from eating really healthy foods. Jane Sen has developed some really fantastic recipes that are suitable for everyone, even if you are planning an important dinner party (*see Chapter 18*).

losing weight

A food intolerance problem can sometimes make it difficult to lose weight, even when you've been eating healthily. **If you've been struggling to shed those extra pounds, you may find that things improve after removing dairy from your diet.** The eating plan outlined here can also help you to lose weight, should you need to do so. Losing weight and keeping it off in the long term doesn't just depend on calorie intake. A better approach is to eat three healthy meals per day with a couple of snacks between meals if you feel peckish. Your diet will consist of lots of healthy fruits and vegetables, good-quality protein and carbohydrate foods, and a small amount of essential fats.

Essential fats can actually help the body shed excess weight. But aim to keep your intake of essential fats quite small; one handful of nuts and seeds and a little bit of oil on salads per day plus a few portions of oily fish a week should be enough. The best oils to use on salads are cold-pressed oils such as olive or sesame.

Avoiding empty calories, such as alcohol and sugary foods, is one of the best ways to achieve healthy and permanent weight loss. The whole of Chapter 12 is devoted to the topic of healthy weight loss so you will find some more tips and ideas there.

eating out and travelling

Eating a dairy-free diet should not be difficult even if you eat out a lot or spend time away from home. Keep a stock of dairy-free substitutes at your workplace. Also have a selection of other healthy foods, such as nuts and seeds, fresh fruit and vegetables, so that you don't have to resort to dairy-containing foods if you feel hungry. If you are travelling, you might need to pack some dairy-free substitutes. I always take a selection of my favourite healthy foods when I'm travelling. It really doesn't take long to sort out what you need. Most hotels provide minibars, so you could even pack things like dairy-free milks. All you need to do is plan ahead by thinking about what foods will be available at your destination and what foods you need to take. Then devise a strategy that suits your needs.

Eating Out

Restaurant food shouldn't pose a problem while you are avoiding dairy. Certain types of cuisine, such as Chinese, Japanese, Thai and Indian (apart from Lassi), rarely use dairy products. You'll also find plenty of dairy-free options in Italian and French restaurants. It's usually easy to spot the recipes that contain dairy, but beware of hidden dairy foods in sauces, soups and even the added milk in mashed potato. If in doubt, ask your waiter. If you are overseas and language is a problem, go for foods that are obviously dairy-free.

8: healing foods

Certain foods are particularly valuable during this phase of the Dairy-free Detox Diet as they have a natural healing effect on your body. Each of these foods works in a slightly different way, so in combination they make a powerful 'healing team' that can help you regain your get up and go and start to strengthen the underlying physical imbalance associated with food intolerance.

flax seeds

These seeds are fantastic powerhouses of different nutrients. They are particularly useful if you have food intolerance because they have a beneficial effect on the whole digestive system. An intolerant food can be quite abrasive on the digestive tract. In contrast, flax seeds are extremely soothing, cooling and healing for the lining of the gut wall. Flax is also a natural and safe way of overcoming constipation. It doesn't have a laxative effect but provides a good source of fibre for the gut.

Flax is a very good source of healthy omega-3 essential fats, which are good for the cardiovascular system, and helpful for healing skin conditions such as eczema (*essential fats are discussed in detail in Chapter 11*).

Flax seeds are available at most health-food shops. They are inexpensive and, as you only need a small amount, will last for ages. If possible, it's best to grind them into a powder as they will be absorbed better (a coffee grinder does this job really well or you could even use a pepper mill). Flax seeds, like all essential fats, can be damaged easily if exposed to light or heat so it's best to store them in the fridge.

Aim to have one tablespoon of ground flax seeds per day (or one tea-spoon of the seeds in their natural form). The easiest way to get them into your diet is to sprinkle them onto your breakfast cereal or mix them into a fruit salad. You can also add them to a fruit smoothie. Jane Sen has pro-vided you with a delicious chocolate pudding recipe that uses flax, so this is well worth creating (*see page 192*).

pineapple

This fruit contains a natural plant enzyme called bromelain, which is helpful for healing the digestive tract and reducing inflammation. It helps the body to make anti-inflammatory substances that are helpful in condi-tions such as eczema, asthma, joint aches and pains and headaches. This natural enzyme also helps break down protein foods, which provides useful support for the whole digestive system. Like all fruits, pineapple is alkaline-forming.

Try to have one or two slices of fresh pineapple each day – before lunch and dinner would be ideal. If you have a juice extractor, you could also make fresh pineapple juice. It tastes absolutely delicious and has an almost creamy texture. It's best to make it fresh rather than buy a carton of juice, as the shop-bought version is unlikely to contain much bromelain. Supplements of bromelain are available if you don't like this fruit.

ginger

This root has a multitude of healing properties. It's an excellent tonic for the digestive system, so is useful for any type of digestive complaint. It has anti-inflammatory properties, which means it can help reduce joint pain and swelling and is a useful natural treatment for headaches. You can get ginger into your diet by using it in cooking, such as adding it to stir-fries, or by making tea. I like to make my own ginger tea but you can buy dried ginger tea in most health food shops.

To Make Ginger Tea

Simply chop up about an inch of fresh ginger root and add it to a saucepan with two cups of water. Bring to the boil and simmer for about five minutes. Sweeten with a teaspoon of honey. It can be made stronger or weaker, depending on the amount of ginger you use. It's an extremely soothing and warming drink during the winter months; I find it really nurturing after coming home at the end of the day when it's cold and dark outside. In the summer you can let the liquid cool and drink it with some crushed ice. If you really don't like the flavour, then you might like to try it in supplement form. Try to have ginger a few times a week at least.

---

vegetable juices

Freshly-prepared vegetable juices are one of the healthiest things you can include in your diet. If you have a juice extractor then you can make your own. Alternatively, bottled juices are widely available, but the fresh version is better for you as it contains plenty of natural enzymes. A juice extractor is not very expensive and it will be a useful addition to your kitchen for many years. I've had mine for about 15 years and it is still going strong!

Carrot juice is particularly beneficial as it can help to heal both the digestive tract and the respiratory system. It's therefore a very good juice to have if you suffer with rhinitis, asthma or frequently get a chesty cough. It is also a good source of the antioxidant betacarotene. Carrot makes a good base juice to which you can add other vegetables. You might like to try carrot with raw beetroot (beet), an excellent combination for detoxing the whole body. If you have fluid retention, then a mix of carrot and celery can be really helpful.

Virtually every vegetable can be juiced. Hard fruits, such as pineapple and apple, are also good to juice. Experiment with different combinations to find those you like best. It's not essential to include vegetable juices in your programme but it will be very beneficial. Try to have one glass of juice each day.

other healing foods

Here are a few other fruits and vegetables that have a naturally healing effect on the digestive tract.

cherries, blueberries and black grapes

These fruits contain powerful antioxidants that help keep the gut wall healthy. The antioxidants they contain have been found to be much more potent than vitamin E. These fruits are widely available during the summer months so try to eat them as often as you can. Blueberries and black grapes are good fruits to use in smoothies as well.

cruciferous vegetables, onions and garlic

The cruciferous vegetables, such as broccoli, cauliflower, cabbage, kale and Brussels sprouts, contain a particular type of fibre that helps to improve the quantity and quality of friendly bacteria in the gut. As discussed below, taking steps to support your digestive flora is important in overcoming food intolerance. These vegetables also contain lots of other important nutrients, including a range of different antioxidants and calcium (especially broccoli).

Onions and garlic are other vegetables to include in your diet regularly as they have natural antifungal and antibacterial properties that also support the health of the friendly bacteria in your gut.

Try to eat cruciferous vegetables, onions and garlic as often as you can. You can rotate the cruciferous vegetables so you don't get bored with eating the same ones. These foods can provoke flatulence. If this happens, it is a signal that your gut flora could be improved somewhat; the flatulence is actually a sign that this is happening. As this is an unpleasant symptom, however, eat smaller quantities of these vegetables to minimize the effect.

nutritional supplements

Certain nutritional supplements are very helpful for overcoming a food intolerance condition. It is possible to deal with food intolerance by simply avoiding the culprit food, eating a healthy diet and choosing foods that have natural healing properties. But you will probably get better results by adding in a few select supplements. For example, the health of friendly bacteria can be improved by eating live soya yoghurt. But this will happen faster if you also take a probiotic supplement, which contains a concentrated source of friendly bacteria.

In the case of essential fats, some people simply cannot metabolize these fats from dietary sources alone (especially if there is a family history of conditions such as eczema and asthma). The only way around this is to take a supplement.

Here are the supplements to take during this first phase of the Dairy-free Detox Diet. You will add another couple during phase two, if there is clear evidence that you do have dairy intolerance:

a good probiotic supplement

In order to reduce the immune system's reaction to certain foods, it is important to strengthen the digestive tract and reduce its tendency to be too leaky. One simple way to do this is to improve the quality and quantity of friendly bacteria that reside in the gut. As discussed earlier, many factors can disrupt the quality of the healthy, friendly bacteria. These include certain medications (such as antibiotics, steroids and the contraceptive pill), stress and a diet high in sugar or alcohol. Eating an intolerant food will also deplete the amount of friendly bacteria in the gut.

You can start to rebalance the flora in your digestive system by taking a supplement of friendly bacteria called a probiotic supplement, which literally means 'pro-life'. Probiotic supplements are available at all health-food shops, so when you go in ask for help in choosing a good brand that contains the *bifido* and *bacillus* cultures (*also see Appendix 5*). As you are avoiding dairy, you need to make sure the supplement is dairy-free, so check the label. Take two tablets per day with a little water (first thing in the morning is best). Keep the supplement in the fridge, as friendly bacteria will die off at room temperature.

essential fatty acids

Many people who have an intolerance to dairy products also have difficulty metabolizing essential fats. Because essential fats are so important to our health, the whole of Chapter 11 is devoted to this topic. Including a supplement of essential fats in your programme is particularly valuable if you have eczema, other skin conditions, asthma, joint aches and pains or premenstrual syndrome.

There are two types of essential fats, omega-6 and omega-3. The active ingredient in omega-6 supplements is gamma linoleic acid (GLA). Evening primrose oil contains about 10 per cent GLA. A good supplementary dose of evening primrose is 1,500 mg per day, which will provide you with 150 mg of GLA. You could spread this evenly through the day (i.e. a 500 mg capsule with breakfast, lunch and dinner). You can also purchase a supplement of pure GLA. If you opt for this approach, aim to take 150 mg per day with food (one capsule usually contains this amount).

If you eat oily fish such as salmon and mackerel at least three times a week, you are probably getting plenty of the omega-3 fats. If you are vegetarian or just don't care for fish, you might like to include an omega-3 fish oil supplement in your programme (note that this is not the same as cod liver oil supplements). A good quality supplement should contain about 300 mg of EPA and 200 mg of DHA (these are substances found in omega-3 fats that you will read about in Chapter 11). Alternatively, there is a marine algae supplement available which provides a good vegetarian source of omega-3 fats. If you are taking any type of blood-thinning medication, talk with your doctor before taking an omega-3 supplement.

multivitamin and multimineral supplements

A multivitamin and a multimineral supplement are an optional, but useful, addition to the programme. **Vitamin and mineral deficiencies are widespread and it is difficult to get absolutely all the nutrients we need from diet alone, even if we eat pretty healthily.** Part of the reason is that the nutrient content of food has declined in recent years due to farming methods that have eroded the levels of minerals in the soil. The nutrient content of organic foods is usually higher, so this is another benefit of choosing these foods.

A multivitamin and a multimineral supplement are beneficial while you are on the Dairy-free Detox Diet, even though the eating plan you will be following is designed to be as rich in nutrients as possible. You will get a little extra support from these supplements that will help correct any nutritional deficiencies you may unknowingly have at the moment. After following the programme for a while, you may decide not to use these supplements anymore.

A multivitamin supplement will supply you with all of the B-vitamins and important antioxidants such as vitamins A, C and E. A multimineral supplement will give you the whole spectrum of important minerals such as zinc, magnesium and iron. It's best to take a separate vitamin and mineral supplement rather than a single supplement that combines both. The vitamin supplement can be taken in the morning with breakfast and will help boost energy during the day. The multimineral supplement is best taken before bed, as minerals such as calcium and magnesium promote deep and restful sleep.

Supplements vary tremendously in terms of quality. It's definitely worth investing in the better quality brands, as these provide a balanced ratio of nutrients and do not use artificial ingredients and unnecessary fillers. *(See Appendix 5 for a selection of companies that make good quality supplements.)*

vitamin c

The eating plan outlined here will provide you with lots of vitamin C. But if you suffer with poor skin, joint aches and pains, respiratory difficulties, headaches or frequent infections then you may benefit from a vitamin C supplement of between 500 mg to 1,000 mg daily. Take this supplement with food, either in the morning or at lunch. Don't take it at the same time as a multimineral supplement. Also, don't use a vitamin C supplement if you are taking the contraceptive pill.

moving on

You now have all the information you need to do the first stage of the Dairy-free Detox Diet. Appendix 3 lists all the dairy-free substitute foods, healing foods and nutritional supplements you need. Once you have completed the two weeks, you can move on to the next chapter which outlines how to interpret any changes in your health symptoms and what to do next.

9: interpreting your results

When you come to the end of the first two weeks on the Dairy-free Detox Diet, you need to look at any changes that have taken place to your health. You might already have quite a clear impression of the effect these last two weeks have had on your health and wellbeing; nevertheless, it is worth spending a couple of minutes completing the following symptom assessment. Then refer back to page 41 and compare your current results with what was recorded on the previous chart. In the final column of this chart you can make a note of the changes. You can use the following scoring system:

✓✓✓ A symptom has completely disappeared or a severe symptom has become mild.

✓✓   A symptom has improved significantly but has not completely disappeared.

✓   A symptom has improved just a little.

◇   No change.

✗   A symptom has become worse.

Post-detox Assessment	None	Mild	Moderate	Severe
Indigestion				
Flatulence				
Constipation				
Diarrhoea				
Abdominal bloating				
Blocked nose				
Chest congestion				
Eczema				
Asthma				
Poor skin				
Headaches				
Migraines				
Fluid retention				
Weight fluctuations				
Joint aches and pains				
Lack of energy				
Tiredness upon waking				
Depression				
Low mood				
Inability to concentrate				
Forgetfulness				
Other:				

you noticed a big improvement (at least a few ✓✓✓ with the remainder mainly ✓✓)

If you noticed a big improvement in your health symptoms during the two-week dairy-free period, this is pretty conclusive evidence that you do have an intolerance to dairy. In this case, you can proceed directly to stage two of the programme. There is no need to do the reintroduction test (*given below*) unless you really want to.

you noticed a reasonably good improvement (mainly ✓✓ and ✓)

This result also suggests that you have a dairy intolerance. Some symptoms such as eczema can take quite a few weeks to respond to the removal of an intolerant food. If you were suffering from digestive problems, a stuffy nose, headaches and/or fluid retention and there has been a reasonable improvement in these conditions, you can move on to stage two. Your remaining symptoms should hopefully continue to improve over the following few weeks. Only do the reintroduction test (*below*) if you feel you need more conclusive evidence.

you noticed a small improvement (mainly ✓)

There are three possible interpretations for this result:

1. You do have dairy intolerance but your particular group of symptoms takes a little longer to respond to eliminating dairy from your diet.
2. You don't have dairy intolerance at all, and the improvement you've experienced is related to the positive changes you've made to your diet during the past two weeks.
3. You may still have dairy intolerance but you are also regularly eating another intolerant food that is involved in your symptoms.

In order to understand a bit more about the relationship between dairy and your health it would be useful for you to do a reintroduction test with dairy, paying particular attention to the pulse test (*see overleaf*). If you do experience a reaction, such as a return of old symptoms or a significant change in your pulse rate, then you can proceed to stage two.

In addition, you might want to take some steps to find out whether or not other foods might be involved in your symptoms. **Other common intolerance culprits are wheat, eggs, soya and the nightshade family – potatoes, tomatoes, aubergines (eggplant) and peppers.** If you kept a food and symptom diary during the past two weeks, have a look to see if you can find any pattern between a particular food and the frequency of a health symptom. For example, if you had eggs on Sunday and your symptoms were worse on Monday or even Tuesday, this suggests you may have a problem with this food. However, if you eat a certain food very often (every day or every other day), it's unlikely that you will be able to notice any pattern between health symptoms and that food.

If you suspect you may be suffering with an intolerance to other foods, one way to proceed is to do another two-week elimination period where you avoid dairy along with the other foods that you suspect may be involved. However, if you decide to avoid other food groups it is *extremely important* to make sure you purchase healthy substitute foods so you are still eating a nutritious, balanced diet and don't run the risk of going hungry. It is still important to eat three meals a day and healthy snacks if you feel peckish. After two weeks you can reintroduce the various foods you are testing, one at a time, leaving three to five days between each reintroduction. You should make a note of any change to your symptoms that occurs after the reintroduction of each food. (*For more on how to carry out a reintroduction test, see page 74.*)

It would probably also be worth consulting a nutritionist and having an ELISA test (*see page 43*). The ELISA test can help you be clear about the foods you are reacting to and the nutritionist can give you lots of advice about creating a healthy diet suitable for your individual needs.

there was hardly any change (mainly ◇ with the occasional ✓)

If you feel the same now as you did two weeks ago and most of your health symptoms have not improved, it is highly unlikely that you have an intolerance to dairy. It is possible that you may be intolerant to other foods. If you suspect this is the case, then read the preceding section for some suggestions on what to do now.

Other factors may also be involved in your symptoms. For example, airborne allergens may be provoking any respiratory problems, or particular detergents or soaps may be implicated in any skin conditions. If you had some emotional upsets or were working very hard during these past two weeks, this might have affected the outcome you have experienced.

To get a clearer idea about the effect of dairy on your wellbeing, you can do the dairy reintroduction test to see if there is any reaction (*see below*). In particular, take note of the pulse test result. If you don't experience any type of reaction, you can be reasonably sure you do not have any problems with dairy.

a particular symptom has become worse (any symptoms you assessed as *x*)

Although it is quite common to feel a bit out of sorts during the first few days after eliminating an intolerant food, this is usually followed by an improvement. More frequent bowel movements should not be interpreted as a sign of things getting worse. For most people, having more bowel movements is a signal that the digestive system is getting healthier. The exception, of course, is frequent diarrhoea, which is not healthy as it means you will not be absorbing the nutrients from your diet adequately.

However, if you have simultaneously made quite a few healthy changes to your diet as well as avoiding dairy during the past two weeks, it may take a while for your body to adjust properly. For example, you may be eating quite a lot more fruits and vegetables than previously. The additional soluble fibre you are getting in your diet could have provoked some bloating, wind or even the odd bout of constipation or diarrhoea. Furthermore, as mentioned in the last chapter, particular vegetables, such as the cruciferous family and onions and garlic, can be quite gas-provoking if your digestive flora are not in tip-top health. You might like to cut back on these foods slightly until your body becomes more used to this new way of eating.

Another interpretation of this result is that your body might have produced a 'cleansing reaction' in response to avoiding dairy foods and following a healthy alkaline-forming diet. Cleansing reaction symptoms are similar to those commonly experienced during a detox that is designed to spring-clean the body. These can be slightly more intense than the usual withdrawal symptoms associated with removing an intolerant food, but they should pass reasonably quickly. A fundamental principle of natural health is that when the body is provided with a breathing space – such as avoiding an intolerant food and eating a nutritious diet – it will take steps to correct any imbalances. **A symptom such as developing a spotty skin could indicate that the body is cleansing and clearing old waste products that have been stored at a cellular level through the skin. Other common cleansing reactions include flu-like symptoms or the occasional bout of diarrhoea. Such symptoms should clear up quite quickly.**

Finally, it is possible that you inadvertently included a new food in your diet to which you have an intolerance and you could be reacting to that. One culprit could be soya products, which do provoke intolerance symptoms in some people. If you think that soya may be a culprit, simply remove it from your diet for about three days. Also, contact your doctor to make sure you are not suffering from any type of illness. Wait until you feel a bit better and then try the dairy reintroduction test (*below*) to determine whether to proceed to stage two.

the reintroduction test

If you are at all unsure about whether or not you are intolerant to dairy, you can now do the reintroduction test. This should provide further evidence of the relationship between dairy and your symptoms. The end of the two-week dairy-free period is a good time to conduct a reintroduction trial. Your system will be quite sensitive to dairy after having avoided this food for two weeks, so the reintroduction test should provide you with a clear result.

You will be using the same test to determine if and when you can reintroduce dairy products into your diet at the end of stage two. This exact same procedure can be used for testing any other food (such as goat's and sheep's milk products). If you are testing multiple foods, you need to allow three to five days between each test.

Conduct the test on a day when you are not too busy and have the opportunity to rest should you need to. For this test use lactose-free milk so that you are testing for dairy intolerance rather than a deficiency of lactase. The procedure for the reintroduction test is as follows:

1. On an empty stomach, drink a glass of milk (or eat a portion of another food you may be testing).
2. Immediately conduct the pulse test (*outlined below*). If the pulse test result is negative and you feel fine over the next few hours, have another portion of the food a few hours later.
3. Continue to monitor how you feel over the next couple of days.

An important short-term signal to look out for is a drop in energy levels, such as feeling suddenly tired or drained. This often happens within a few hours of an intolerant food being reintroduced into the diet. Another common signal that suggests that intolerance is present is if you suddenly feel hot and sweaty or unnaturally cold. Again, these symptoms usually occur within a few hours of consuming an intolerant food. Also notice whether there is any recurrence or worsening of health symptoms, particularly changes in your digestive system during the next few days. Any combination of these signals suggests that you are intolerant to the particular food you are testing. The pulse test provides additional evidence.

the pulse test

The pulse test is another way of finding out whether or not a particular food is provoking an intolerance reaction. It is very easy to do:

1. Sit down and relax for five minutes and then take your pulse before eating the food you are testing.
2. Eat the food and, after about 10 minutes, measure your pulse again.
3. Wait another 20 minutes and take a final pulse measurement.
4. During the 30 minutes it takes to do this test, it is best to remain seated

and relaxed. Don't rush around or watch any television programmes that are overstimulating (an exciting movie will obviously increase your pulse rate).

A significant change in your pulse rate (either increasing or decreasing) suggests that you are intolerant to the particular food you are testing. A significant change is in the region of 15–20 beats per minute. This might occur after 10 minutes or after 30 minutes, or both. Usually the pulse goes up but a significant reduction should also be interpreted as an important result.

The pulse test is not always totally accurate. Therefore the result should be used in combination with any changes you experience in your symptoms over the next two days. For example, if your pulse does not react but you experience a recurrence of symptoms, the latter is a stronger signal that intolerance is present.

10: what next?

Now you've found out what's causing your symptoms, it's time to move on to the second stage of the Dairy-free Detox Diet. Here, you will follow a natural healing plan to strengthen the body systems involved in food intolerance.

It is best to follow this stage of the programme for three months. You need to continue to avoid all dairy foods for the time being so you don't trigger the immune response that could result in your symptoms returning. At the end of the programme, you can choose to start eating dairy again, should you wish to do so. Many people find that they no longer react to a previously intolerant food once they have cut it out for about three months and taken steps to support the health of the digestive tract and other body systems.

what to expect

This part of the programme builds on what you have already been doing. The eating plan remains pretty much the same, although there are a few additional suggestions. Some extra nutritional supplements are also recommended as they are specifically designed to help the digestive system. These supplements are all based on naturally occurring ingredients found in food, but in a more concentrated form. If you don't like taking supplements, don't worry. You will still get good results just by following the dietary advice.

The health benefits you have already experienced should continue during the next few weeks. The body has an amazing ability to heal itself and restore lost vitality and health. What you are doing on the Dairy-free Detox Diet is creating a space – by avoiding an intolerant food and eating a nutritious, balanced diet – for the body to do this job.

When the body is going through a period of self-healing, you may find that symptoms you haven't experienced for a long time make a temporary return. Suzanna found that her joint aches and pains improved greatly after she eliminated the foods to which she had an intolerance. She continued to avoid these foods, but a month later she noticed that she had a small amount of eczema on her arms. As she hadn't experienced eczema since she was a child, her initial reaction was that something was going wrong. However, she stuck with her eating plan and the eczema vanished within a few days. She also noticed that her energy levels improved greatly the week after the bout of eczema.

This type of phenomenon is very common when working with natural approaches to healing. Some people experience symptoms of what appears to be a cold or flu but may actually be the body ridding itself of excess mucus that it has been storing for some time. It's important to follow your own judgement when monitoring your health. If you are concerned about any health symptom then go and see your doctor. But with minor problems such as cold-like symptoms, it's best to wait for a few days before resorting to medication.

the importance of the digestive system

We have already looked at the relationship between the digestive tract and food intolerance. Here is some more information about why it's important to strengthen this system.

Conditions such as eczema might initially seem to be completely unrelated to what's going on in the digestive tract, but we nutritionists see it differently. In fact, as a profession, we're all somewhat obsessed with the health of the digestive system! This is because **what happens in the digestive system influences literally every aspect of our**

**health and wellbeing. If we can take steps to support the diges-
tive system, our overall health is likely to improve as well.**

The digestive tract is the only direct point of contact between food and the body. The gut wall provides a protective barrier that stops foreign sub-stances (such as microbes, toxins and partially-digested food molecules) from getting into the body where they could cause damage. A complex set of immune-related functions occurs in the gut, which in turn influ-ences immune reactions throughout the body.

leaky gut

Modern life places a great deal of strain on the digestive system. The typi-cal Western diet simply doesn't provide the right type of nutrients to keep the digestive system in tip-top health. As you've already seen, food intol-erance puts even more strain on the digestive system. In most cases of food intolerance, the gut has become too 'leaky', which means it is able to let through unwanted substances. The nutritional approaches discussed below can help reduce gut leakiness, which will in turn reduce the likeli-hood of intolerance-related health symptoms.

A leaky gut is also associated with other problems. It can, for instance, impair our ability to absorb nutrients from food. Minerals are absorbed across the gut wall by certain carrier molecules, a sort of taxi service at a molecular level. These carrier molecules are damaged when the gut becomes too leaky, meaning that mineral deficiencies are much more likely.

Let's first have a look at the particular nutritional supplements that can support the health of the digestive system. Eating guidelines for stage two of the Dairy-free Detox Diet are discussed next.

making friends with our friendly bacteria

One of the easiest yet most effective ways to improve the health of the digestive system is to take steps to increase the level of friendly bacteria that reside in the gut. You have already started to do this by taking a probiotic supplement. These friendly bacteria are extremely important to our health. They are particularly important for dealing with a food intolerance condition because they help to heal the gut wall and also have a direct effect on the immune response associated with intolerance symptoms.

In days gone by, our diet contained *several thousand times* more bacteria than it does today. The food storage methods used by our ancestors resulted in a natural fermentation process that provided the right conditions for these bacteria to develop. Having bacteria in food doesn't sound like something we would either want or need. But the bacteria that used to occur naturally in food were primarily strains of the healthy, friendly flora that provide lots of health-promoting benefits for the digestive tract and the whole body.[1] Modern food processing and storage methods mean that we no longer get sufficient quantities of these friendly bacteria in our diet. This is believed to be an important factor in the rise of conditions such as eczema, asthma and food allergy and intolerance.[2]

There are hundreds of different strains of bacteria residing in our digestive system but not all of them offer health-promoting benefits. The 'friendly' variety (the *bifido* and *bacillus* strains) are good for us whereas others (the bacteroids) promote problems such as excessive flatulence, bloating and other digestive disturbances. Factors such as poor diet, stress and certain medications (antibiotics, steroids and the contraceptive pill) will deplete the friendly bacteria and allow the less healthy strains to proliferate along with other unwanted substances, such as yeast.

Did you know?

Our friendly bacteria are established from the moment we are born. A natural birth and breast-feeding help to establish the right balance of healthy bacteria, whereas a delivery via caesarean section, although necessary in certain circumstances, disrupts this natural process, as does bottle-feeding.[3]

The friendly bacteria help to keep the gut wall healthy. They are also beneficial to a whole host of immune-related functions within the body. They help the body to control inflammation within the gut and within the body as a whole, thereby helping with symptoms such as:

- eczema
- rhinitis
- headaches
- joint aches and pains

Taking a probiotic supplement can therefore help to reduce gut leakiness[4] and immune-related symptoms associated with both food intolerance and food allergy.[5,6] Friendly bacteria also have lots of other important jobs to perform:

- they manufacture certain vitamins (some B-vitamins and vitamin K)
- they help the digestive tract absorb minerals, such as calcium and magnesium
- they help lower blood cholesterol

To continue the good work you're doing to improve the level of friendly bacteria in your gut, aim to take your probiotic supplement for another six weeks or so. You can reduce the level to just one tablet (rather than two) per day.

FOS: food for your friendly bacteria

You can enhance what you are doing to re-establish a good balance of digestive flora by also taking a supplement of FOS. This supplement is not essential, but it will help to create a healthy level of gut flora faster than just taking the probiotic supplement on its own.[7] Like probiotics, FOS helps the body to absorb minerals such as calcium, magnesium and zinc.[8]

FOS stands for fructo-oligo-saccharides. It is a naturally occurring substance derived from certain vegetables such as the cruciferous vegetables and asparagus. FOS provides 'food' for your friendly bacteria, helping them to grow and flourish. In addition, FOS provides extra healthy fibre for the digestive tract, thereby helping to promote regular bowel movements.

FOS is available as a powder or in capsule form. The powder is very versatile as it can be sprinkled onto cereals or mixed into water or other drinks. It has a slightly sweet taste. FOS can be somewhat gas producing until the flora in the digestive tract starts to become more balanced. Therefore, if you decide to take this supplement, start off slowly. Start with half a teaspoon a day and gradually build up to 1–2 teaspoons. Take it either on an empty stomach or with a small meal such as breakfast.

glutamine: nourishment for the digestive tract

Glutamine is a wonderful tonic for the digestive system that can also help to heal the gut wall. It is an amino acid (protein) that is naturally occurring in food. The body can also make glutamine, but if the digestive system is under par, levels of this nutrient may be deficient. Glutamine provides 'fuel' for the cells of the digestive system (and certain lymphatic cells), helping them to regenerate. It can also help to reduce cravings for sugar, stimulants and alcohol and is very useful if you are suffering from fatigue.

You can buy glutamine in either capsule or powder form. The powder form is easy to take as it is tasteless and mixes easily with water. A good supplemental dose is about four grams (equivalent to one teaspoon of the powder) per day. You can take it either with food or on an empty stomach.

your supplement plan

The following chart outlines the suggested supplement plan for this stage of the programme. You might not need the omega-3 supplement if you frequently eat oily fish. As discussed in Chapter 8, the multivitamin, multimineral and vitamin C supplements are optional. The 'duration' stated in the chart starts from the beginning of stage two. You can continue to take the omega supplements, multivitamin, multimineral and vitamin C in the longer term.

supplement plan for stage two

Supplement	Amount per day	Duration
Probiotics	1 tablet	6 weeks
FOS	1–2 teaspoons (5–10g)	6 weeks
Glutamine	1 teaspoon (4g)	6 weeks
Omega-6	150mg GLA	3 months
Omega-3	300mg EPA, 200mg DHA	3 months
Multivitamin	1 tablet with breakfast	3 months
Vitamin C	500–1,000mg	3 months
Multimineral	1 tablet before bed	3 months

eating guidelines for stage two

The same dietary principles you were introduced to in Chapter 7 should be followed during phase two of the programme, and indeed in the longer term as well. Now you are pretty sure that you do have a food intolerance condition, you should avoid certain foods that don't support the digestive system.

coffee

One culprit is coffee, including decaffeinated, which can irritate the gut wall. Therefore, it's best to avoid coffee. Instead, drink herb teas and the occasional cup of black tea. Dandelion coffee has a similar taste to regular coffee so this is an alternative you may like to try. Dandelion root is an excellent tonic for the liver and can help the body to rid itself naturally of excess fluid. Dandelion coffee is available in instant form, but this product usually contains dairy. Instead, go for the natural root and grind up the amount you need into a powder. Steep in boiling water in a cafetière for five minutes and then add soya milk and sweetener to taste.

sugary foods and alcohol

These can disrupt the balance of friendly bacteria in the gut so it is wise to keep your intake low. It's even better to avoid them completely if you can. Avoiding coffee and reducing alcohol and sugary foods is also helpful for your liver.

spicy food

Food containing chilli, cayenne or paprika should be eaten only once in a while as the spices can increase gut permeability.[9]

wheat

Wheat, especially wheat bran, can also be abrasive to the digestive system. You don't have to avoid wheat totally, but it's better to keep your intake to moderate levels and to rotate it with other grains. If you have a wheat bran cereal for breakfast (All Bran or Bran Flakes), experiment with alternatives, such as porridge mixed with added oat bran or other grains like buckwheat.

healthy eating

The other guidelines given in Chapter 7 should help you create a balanced, nutritious, healthy diet:

- eat plenty of fruits and vegetables
- choose good-quality protein and carbohydrate foods and modest amounts of essential fats
- keep the amount of processed foods in your diet to a minimum

It's also important to include plenty of variety in your diet. Don't eat the same foods every day. This helps ensure you are getting the full spectrum of nutrients you need and also makes it less likely that you will develop intolerance problems to other foods.

You can continue to eat the healing foods discussed in Chapter 8. As you saw, these foods have a highly beneficial effect on the digestive tract. They are also good for the liver and lymphatic system, which are overworked when food intolerance is present. It's good to continue having some flax seeds every day. Try to eat the other foods as frequently as possible, rotating them from day-to-day. To remind you, these healing foods are:

- pineapple
- the cruciferous vegetables (broccoli, cabbage, cauliflower, Brussels sprouts, kale)
- black cherries
- blueberries
- ginger
- onions
- garlic

All these foods contain other nutrients that are beneficial for your liver, which will have been working extra hard to deal with a food intolerance condition. If you are making your own fresh vegetable juices, continue having a glass every day. Finally, don't forget to keep drinking plenty of water.

You'll find some other important dietary guidelines in Chapters 13 and 14, which discuss how to get sufficient calcium and other important minerals, and dietary strategies to look after your bones.

testing non-dairy milks, yoghurts and cheeses

Christine had an intolerance to dairy foods. She found they provoked symptoms such as digestive problems, migraines and a stuffy nose. After avoiding dairy for two weeks, these symptoms cleared up. She then introduced some goat's and sheep's milk products and found that she remained symptom-free.

Quite a few people who have an intolerance to dairy can tolerate goat's and sheep's milk products. You might be able to as well, but it is best to go through a reintroduction test first, should you wish to include these foods in your diet.

Follow the procedure for reintroducing foods described in Chapter 9. Do the pulse test as well. With goat's and sheep's milk products, start off by testing milk and yoghurt. Live yoghurt made from goat's or sheep's milk provides a good source of friendly bacteria. If you are fine with these, progress on to goat's and/or sheep's cheese. Provided that you don't react to your first portion, have a second portion on the same day. Then wait for three to five days, during which time you should look out for any changes in your health symptoms. Some symptoms such as eczema can take more than a few days to emerge. If you do notice a decline in your health over the next couple of weeks, remove these foods from your diet.

after three months

By this stage you should have experienced many improvements to your overall health and wellbeing. You can now test to see whether or not you can include dairy into your diet again, should you wish to do so. The process for reintroducing dairy is similar to the one you used to introduce goat's and sheep's products. Start with milk and yoghurt. Wait at least three to five days and observe any effects. If you are okay with milk and yoghurt, you can test with cheese. The pulse test is unlikely to give you useful information at this point as you have avoided dairy for some time. **Not everybody can reintroduce an intolerant food at this point. Some people might take a lot longer to reduce their reactivity. Everybody is unique, so it's best to follow the guidance your body gives you.**

reintroducing dairy

If you do opt to eat dairy products in the longer term, low-fat milk and live yoghurt are much better for you than cheese, cream, butter and similar dairy products. As you've seen, cheese, especially high-protein cheeses, has a strong acid-forming effect on the body. Milk and yoghurt are much better in this respect, and live yoghurt will provide healthy friendly bacteria. Even though you might no longer react to dairy products, it is still wise to keep your intake of dairy foods low. If you fall into a pattern of eating a large amount of a food to which you have had an intolerance, your body could soon start to react to that food again.[10]

lactose intolerance

Although you may no longer react to dairy protein, there is still the issue of lactose intolerance. The friendly bacteria in live yoghurt pre-digest the lactose, so people with lactose intolerance can often tolerate this food. Certain cheeses, such as Swiss cheese, only contain small amounts of lactose.

An easy way of finding out whether or not a dairy food contains lactose is to check the label for carbohydrate content. With respect to dairy products, carbohydrate and lactose are the same thing. Therefore, if the label on the cheese says 'negligible carbohydrate', it is virtually lactose-free.

11: why fats are essential

Earlier on, we looked at why you could benefit from supplements of both omega-3 and omega-6 fats. This chapter explains why these fats are so important. It also discusses how a high intake of dairy foods can prevent the body using these healthy fats properly.

If you suffer with any of the following, it is highly likely that you have a deficiency of essential fats:

- eczema
- dry skin
- joint aches and pains
- premenstrual syndrome

Dietary fat has got a bad name for itself over the past few years. Many people who are trying to lose weight are fat phobic and fret about putting even the tiniest drop of oil onto their salad. But this really is a very unhealthy approach. **If you want to have shiny hair, glowing skin, a positive mood, a healthy heart and much, much more, you need to make sure you are getting an adequate intake of essential fats.**

how the body uses essential fats

Fats are either saturated or unsaturated. Animal products (cheese, butter, meat and eggs) contain high amounts of saturated fats. Unsaturated fats are found mainly in nuts, seeds, oils and fish and they are classified as either monounsaturated or polyunsaturated.

Olive oil is primarily a monounsaturated fat. This type of fat is not considered essential as the body can convert other fats into this form. But nevertheless olive oil is a very healthy type of fat to eat.

Polyunsaturated fats are classed as essential because the nutrients they provide can only be derived from our diet. The exception to this rule is arachidonic acid, which is the polyunsaturated fat found in dairy products and meat. This is not essential as the body can make whatever amount of arachidonic acid it needs from other polyunsaturated fats.

Although it is important for us to keep saturated fats to a minimum in our diets, most of us would benefit from increasing our intake of essential fats. These fats play a role in a multitude of vital bodily functions including:

- looking after the heart and cardiovascular system
- balancing hormones
- helping the brain to work properly

People who have an intolerance to dairy often also have difficulty metabolizing essential fats. It is therefore worth making sure that your essential fat intake is properly balanced. **Conditions such as premenstrual syndrome, eczema and other skin problems often improve once steps are taken to get the right balance of fats in the diet.**

the two types of essential fats

Essential fatty acids come in two forms, omega-3 and omega-6.

omega-3

There are three forms of omega-3 fats. Some start life as ALA (alpha-linolenic acid). Flax seeds, for example, are high in ALA. When we eat flax seeds, the body converts the ALA into both EPA (eicosapentanoic acid) and DHA (docosahexaenoic acid).

When we eat oily fish, we get a direct source of EPA and DHA. This is because the fish eat plankton, a great source of ALA, and this has already been converted to the other forms by the time we eat it.

omega-6

Omega-6 comes in two forms, linoleic acid and arachidonic acid. Arachidonic acid has some important functions but too much of it can disrupt hormones, increase blood clotting and provoke pain and swelling (*see Chapter 3*). As the body can make arachidonic acid directly from linoleic acid, the former doesn't need to be supplied from the diet. (*For more on how the body converts essential fatty acids, see Chapter 16.*) Food sources of these fats are listed below.

---

good sources of essential fatty acids

Omega-3 **EPA and DHA**	Omega-6 **Linoleic Acid**
Halibut	Sunflower seeds/oil
Salmon	Sesame seeds/oil
Mackerel	Pumpkin seeds/oil
Herring	Corn oil
Tuna	Soy beans
Cod	Safflower oil

ALA	**Arachidonic Acid**
Flax seeds	Dairy products
Walnuts	Meat
Pumpkin seeds	
Canola oil*	
Soy beans and soy bean oil*	

* Often found in unhealthy hydrogenated form in processed foods

---

essential fats in our diet

The ratio of omega-3 to omega-6 fatty acids in the diet has become unbalanced during the past century. The diets of the hunter-gatherer tribes (400,000–45,000 years ago) consisted of an equal balance of omega-3 to omega-6. Our ancestors derived their essential fats from wild plants, animals and fish. Wild animals would consume plants and seeds that were high in omega-3 and thus would have high concentrations of these fats in their flesh. However, modern farming methods and the widespread use of vegetable oils in food manufacturing have resulted in a significant decline of omega-3 fats in the food supply and a simultaneous increase in the level of omega-6.

It is widely accepted that to promote health and wellbeing, the best ratio of omega-3 to omega-6 should be between 1:1 to 1:2. However, modern diets usually consist of only 1mg of omega-3 for every 10mg of omega-6. Some diets provide an unbalanced ratio as high as 1:30. However, it's unlikely that the high intake of omega-6 comes from healthier options, such as seeds and unrefined seed oils. Rather, the imbalance towards omega-6 comes from inferior sources such as trans fats that are widely used in processed foods and vegetable spreads (*see below*), and the arachidonic acid found in dairy products and meat.

health benefits of essential fats

It is definitely worthwhile getting sufficient essential fats and making sure that they are in balance, as the omegas are truly wonder foods. Here are a few of the health-promoting benefits of these nutrients.

EPA can significantly reduce the risk of heart disease. It does this by improving the balance of good to bad cholesterol and lowering the level of fats in the blood. It also encourages the body to reduce the stickiness of blood cells and decreases levels of lipoprotein (a), both major risk factors for cardiovascular disease.[1] On the other hand, the arachidonic acid found in dairy foods and meat increases the stickiness of blood cells, raising the risk of blood clots and hence heart disease.

DHA plays a vital role when it comes to intelligence and proper brain and nerve function. The brain is 60 per cent fat and every nerve cell in the brain contains both DHA and arachidonic acid. People with low levels of DHA in their diets perform less well in intelligence tests than those with high DHA. Supplementing with omega-3 fats and GLA (*see below*) have led to improvements in the reading ability of people with dyslexia.

The nervous system relies on sufficient levels of DHA for proper functioning. Diseases of the nervous system, such as multiple sclerosis, can be supported by an adequate intake of omega-3. Seventy per cent of brain cells are formed while the foetus is developing inside the mother's womb so it is vital that sufficient omega fats are consumed during pregnancy. These fats also contribute to the development of the nervous system and the eyes. As omega-3 fats are usually less abundant in the diet than omega-6, it may be advisable to take a fish oil supplement during pregnancy.

A lack of omega-3 has been associated with depression and low mood. Omega-3 has also proved useful in treating people with bipolar disease (manic depression). There is also strong evidence that this essential fat can help to protect against cancer of the digestive system (oesophagus, stomach and colon). Omega-3, along with other vital nutrients such as selenium and vitamin E, may also protect the health of the prostate gland and reduce the risk of breast cancer.

Essential Fats and Weight Loss

People often avoid fats when they are trying to lose weight. Although it is true that fats are higher in calories than other types of food, the essential fatty acids, especially the omega-3 variety, actually promote weight loss. One scientific study followed two groups of people over a period of eight weeks. Total daily calorie intake was the same for everyone. The only difference between the groups was that one group consumed oily fish a couple of times a week. The fish-eating group lost on average two kilos more by the end of the study than the non-fish-eating group. The reason for this is that omega-3 fats support the proper functioning of the metabolic rate, thereby helping weight loss.

The omega-6 fats (not arachidonic acid) play an important role in a variety of conditions. A deficiency of omega-6 fats is associated with:

- depression
- premenstrual syndrome
- skin problems such as eczema
- attention deficit disorder
- dry skin
- dry eyes
- dull, lifeless hair

PMS symptoms such as bloating, sugar cravings and irritability can all improve once the right type of omega-6 fats are included in the diet. Health conditions for which the omega fats have been found helpful are given below.

---

health problems that can be helped with essential fatty acids

Omega-3	Omega-6
High cholesterol, blood fats & stickiness	Skin problems, eczema
Heart disease	Dry eyes
Depression	Premenstrual syndrome
Inability to concentrate, forgetfulness	Excessive thirst
Hyperactivity	Dull hair and dandruff
Skin problems	Depression
Foetal development during pregnancy	
Multiple sclerosis	
Dyslexia	

powerful prostaglandins

Another function of omega fats is to produce prostaglandins. These are hormone-like substances that live only for a few seconds, yet have a dramatic impact on our health. Omega-3 fats and the oils and seeds from the omega-6 family produce anti-inflammatory prostaglandins that can help to alleviate conditions such as:

- rheumatoid arthritis
- migraines
- eczema
- hay fever
- asthma
- PMS

They can also help to balance blood sugar problems, which will reduce sugar cravings, mood swings and fatigue. On the other hand, too much arachidonic acid, the omega-6 fat found in dairy products and meat, can aggravate all these conditions. (*For more about omega fats and prostaglandins, see Chapter 15.*)

throw away those vegetable spreads

Have you noticed that we no longer see those adverts on TV that tell us to purchase vegetable spreads because they are 'good for your heart'? **Although vegetable oils are healthy, vegetable spreads have been found to be even more damaging to your heart than saturated fats!** This fact has been known for quite some time but it has taken many years for manufacturers to stop bombarding us with these misleading promotions. Presumably, as consumers became more aware of the problem, manufacturers finally had no option but to withdraw their claims.

unhealthy trans fats

The reason why margarine and vegetable spreads are so unhealthy is that they contain trans fats (also referred to as hydrogenated or partially hydrogenated fats). Trans fats are formed during the process of converting an oil into a solid, which distorts and damages the oil at the molecular level. Trans fats are a relatively new addition to our diet and the body basically does not know how to use the unfamiliar chemical molecules found in these products. It is estimated that approximately 25 per cent of total fat intake (including saturates) in the average diet comes from these unhealthy trans fats.

It is now recognized that trans fats pose a number of health risks. As mentioned, they inhibit the conversion of omega fats by the body, so even if there are plenty of these good fats in the diet, the body is unable to use them properly. Further, there is a vast body of evidence that trans fats increase the level of LDLs (the bad cholesterol) and suppress HDLs (good cholesterol) in the blood. Saturated fats also create the same effect, but trans fats have twice as much impact in this respect.

Harvard researchers suggest that, at the most conservative estimate, trans fats are accountable for *30,000 unnecessary deaths per year* from heart disease in the United States alone.[2] Trans fats can also get into brain cells where they replace the omega-3 DHA molecules, which will negatively affect mental functioning.

Trans fats are damaged at the molecular level, which means that they are a source of free radicals in the diet. Free radicals are known to be associated with an increased risk of cancer. It has also been estimated that replacing trans fats with natural liquid oils could reduce the intake of adult-onset diabetes in the United States by as much as 40 per cent.[3]

Thus, trans fats are without a doubt particularly terrible to our health and we should definitely avoid them. **Vegetable spreads that have not been hydrogenated are available; the best place to find them is in the health-food shop. Nut or seed butters are a good alternative to vegetable spreads. You could look out for almond, cashew and pumpkin seed butters. Tahini can also be spread onto toast or crackers.**

Although the most obvious source of trans fats is vegetable spreads, they are also used extensively in food manufacturing as vegetable shortening. Hence, many cookies, cakes, popcorn and similar processed foods can contain significant quantities of them. Dried milk powders and products made with them also contain trans fats. The best strategy is to read labels when you are out shopping. If you see the words 'hydrogenated' or 'partially hydrogenated', then put the product back on the shelf. This might be time consuming, but the benefits are definitely worth it.

Frying food, especially deep-frying, also generates trans fats. Therefore, it's best to limit your intake of foods such as doughnuts, French fries and the like, plus avoid buying processed foods that involve deep-frying, such as crisps. For shallow-frying at home, use a little olive oil. This monounsaturated fat is much less liable to be damaged by heat.

getting our essential fats in balance

omega-3

A good intake of both EPA and DHA can be achieved by eating three to four portions of oily fish per week. Salmon and sardines are excellent as they also contain lots of calcium (*see Chapter 13*). Try to buy fish that has been caught from clean waters as they can become contaminated with environmental toxins.

If you don't like fish, you may wish to take a fish oil supplement. A good quality supplement will contain at least 300mg of EPA and 200mg of DHA. Omega-3 fats are not toxic so it's safe to take these in higher amounts. If you are taking any form of blood-thinning medication, have a chat with your doctor before taking omega-3 supplements.

The flax seeds you have been eating also provide omega-3 fats. Walnuts are another good vegetarian source of these fats. But the conversion by the body of the ALA from flax and other vegetable sources into EPA and DHA is not that efficient. Therefore, if you are vegetarian you may still be low in omega-3, even if you are consuming these foods. There is a marine algae supplement available which provides a useful strategy for vegetarians to boost their omega-3 intake.

omega-6

We definitely need sufficient omega-6 in our diets for all of the health benefits described above. However, this is the first time in history that we have consumed such a high amount of omega-6 and there is some concern that very high levels may not be healthy. The key is to try to get both omega-3 and omega-6 into balance. For most of us, this means cutting back on our use of vegetable oils and vegetable spreads, and avoiding the omega-6 found in trans fats. You really don't need much of these fats to meet your daily requirements. One tablespoon per day of sunflower oil or one handful of seeds will suffice. Personally, I prefer to use olive oil on salads and for cooking and get my omega-6 from eating seeds.

supplements

You can continue to take the omega-3 and omega-6 supplements in the longer term. In addition to supplements in capsule form, two products to look out for are *Udo's Choice* or *Essential Balance*. Both of these products provide a balanced ratio of omega-3 and omega-6. They are available as oils that can be easily added to foods and juices. One tablespoon of these oils per day is a good dose.

getting fats into balance

Avoid	Reduce	Increase
Trans fats	Saturated fats	Flax
Deep fried food	Arachidonic acid	Walnuts and other nuts
	Vegetable oils	Olive oil
	Vegetable spreads*	Oily fish
		Pumpkin seeds
		Sesame seeds
		Sunflower seeds

* Only eat vegetable spreads if they are unhydrogenated

get plenty of antioxidants

We store essential fats in the body, including the cells of the brain and nervous system, where they can also be damaged. Toxic substances such as cigarette smoke and environmental pollution can cause havoc with these fats at a cellular level. It is therefore important that our diet contains plenty of antioxidant nutrients, especially vitamin E whose job it is to protect fat molecules. Other antioxidant nutrients include vitamin C, betacarotene, zinc and selenium. The eating plan you have been following on the Dairy-free Detox Diet is high in fruits, vegetables and whole foods, so you will be getting plenty of antioxidant nutrients.

Oxygen, light and heat will damage oils and seeds so you need to store them carefully. It's best to keep seeds in the fridge and to store oils in a cool cupboard where they won't be exposed to direct sunlight. A useful tip is to pierce a vitamin E capsule and add this to the bottle of oil. This will help to protect the oil from oxidative damage (it leaves no taste). Buy good quality oils (cold pressed are best) and don't use them after the expiry date. Also, it's best not to fry foods with the omega-6 oils such as sunflower, safflower or sesame. Instead, use a little olive oil; as this is monounsaturated, it is less prone to heat damage. You can add a teaspoon of sesame oil to stir-fries after cooking so that you still get the flavour.

12: food intolerance and weight loss

A food intolerance condition can make it harder to lose weight, even when following a reduced-calorie diet. This chapter looks at the link between food intolerance and body weight and provides healthy strategies for losing any excess weight you may have.

fluid retention

As you've already seen, food intolerance is often associated with bloating and fluid retention. Excess fluid can be particularly stubborn to shift until the culprit food is removed from the diet. Many people are pleasantly surprised to discover that they have lost quite a few pounds in the first week or two after removing an intolerant food from their diet. Once the conditions are right, the body can remove excess fluid quite quickly. In addition to the changes we notice on the bathroom scales, eliminating excess fluid can make us look and feel much better.

food cravings

Another way food intolerance can make weight loss more difficult is by provoking cravings. Cravings for the intolerant food are believed to affect about 50 per cent of people with food intolerance. As these cravings are physical in nature, even the strongest willpower in the world can succumb to them. These cravings can make any attempts to follow a weight-loss plan particularly difficult. As you may have already noticed, these cravings usually subside after a few days of avoiding the offending food.

diets don't work

There are literally hundreds of different diet plans available, but how many of these approaches actually work in the long run is questionable. The words I associate with 'diet' include deprivation, hard work, hunger pangs, willpower battles and feeling awful. **Let's face it, if diets really did work then the multibillion-dollar diet industry wouldn't exist and obesity rates would not be steadily increasing.**

I don't believe that you have to count calories or use an excessive amount of willpower to battle hunger pangs in order to reach your ideal weight. If you need to lose weight, the Dairy-free Detox Diet is a great eating plan to help you achieve your goal in a healthy and sustainable way. This chapter outlines certain key principles that will help you lose any excess weight in a healthy fashion and to keep it off in the longer term.

The approach outlined here consists of eating three healthy meals per day plus a couple of snacks if you need them. In fact, you are encouraged to eat whenever you feel genuinely hungry, which means that the level of willpower you need is virtually zero. By following these principles you should be able to lose weight at a steady pace, usually at a rate of 1–3 pounds per week. Losing weight slowly increases the likelihood that weight loss will be permanent (releasing excess fluid can result in quite a large amount of weight loss within a short period, but this is different to shedding fat tissue).

ending cravings for good

Following a very restricted calorie diet or skipping meals doesn't usually help us to achieve our ideal weight in the long term. We might be able to follow this type of diet for a short while but sooner or later we get so

hungry that our willpower fails and we succumb to that piece of chocolate cake. And, after falling victim to cravings, it's usual to overcompen-
sate by eating too much, which means that we end up even heavier than
before we started. Even if we don't overeat, however, we may still gain
weight quite quickly when we end a highly restrictive diet plan. This is
because we have inadvertently created the right conditions for the body
to convert the food we eat into fat tissue very easily.

stabilizing energy levels

There is an easy way to avoid these problems. **The most effective way
of achieving permanent and healthy weight loss is to make sure
you follow an eating plan that will keep your energy levels stable.**
This approach provides two extremely important benefits:

1. It will really help to reduce cravings, which means you are much more
   likely to stick with your weight-loss goals and avoid indulging in foods
   that will stop you from losing weight.
2. It will totally support your metabolism so that weight loss happens easily
   and without risk of a rebound effect. In other words, you will lose weight
   without ever feeling starving and will also be able to maintain your new
   weight in the long term.

Energy slumps in the middle of the afternoon, suddenly feeling irritable
or depressed for no apparent reason and cravings for sugary or carbohydrate foods can indicate that your blood sugar balance has become disrupted. Weight fluctuations can also suggest that this mechanism needs
some support. A food intolerance problem can disrupt the delicate mechanisms that control blood sugar and metabolism. Once the culprit food
is removed, these symptoms can stabilize very quickly as long as you
are following an eating plan that helps balance your blood sugar levels.

However, many people suffer with a blood sugar imbalance even
when there isn't a food intolerance condition. The typical modern diet
simply does not do a good job of keeping our blood sugar and energy

levels balanced. Other factors such as stress and a high intake of caffeine also perpetuate the problem.

As well as being the most effective way of losing weight, making sure we choose foods that help keep our energy levels stable will pay big dividends to our health and wellbeing. It helps to create more physical energy, balanced emotions and a clear and focused mind. Furthermore, most symptoms associated with premenstrual syndrome usually stabilize once this type of eating pattern is followed (PMS is often also related to magnesium deficiency, and magnesium is also important for blood sugar balance).

eating the right carbs

The Dairy-free Detox Diet you have been following recommends certain types of carbohydrate foods that will keep your energy levels balanced and help you to lose weight, should you need to. This chapter explains why these types of carbohydrate are important.

Carbohydrates are an essential part of a healthy diet. When we eat carbohydrates they are eventually converted into glucose, the body's favourite source of energy. But carbohydrate foods differ significantly in terms of how they are handled by the body. Some carbohydrates are converted into glucose very quickly. These types of carbohydrate can make us gain weight in two ways:

1. Releasing a lot of glucose into the bloodstream quickly results in blood sugar levels becoming higher than they should be. This is a potentially dangerous situation, so certain mechanisms spring into action to bring this level down. As this excess glucose has to go somewhere, the body will often store it as fat.

2. Eating a diet containing carbohydrates that release their energy very quickly creates conditions that prompt us to eat much more food than we need to. This happens because of the quick rise and fall in blood sugar levels that happen after eating fast-releasing carbohydrates. A fall in

blood sugar levels will send specific hunger signals to the brain. We will feel hungry again quite quickly after eating a fast-releasing carbohydrate food, often within an hour or two. These hunger pangs will propel us to eat extra food, especially high-sugar snacks such as cookies or cakes, which definitely don't fit in with our weight-loss plans.

the glycaemic index

The rate at which different carbohydrates release their energy is calculated in the glycaemic index (GI). Foods are ranked relative to glucose, which has a standard score of 100. The higher the score, the faster the food is turned into glucose. High and low-GI foods create substantially different effects on how we feel and on our weight. For example, puffed rice breakfast cereals have a high GI score (87), meaning they are converted into glucose very quickly. Eating puffed rice for breakfast will usually result in us feeling very hungry by 11am so we reach for the cookie jar to replenish our energy levels. On the other hand, porridge (which has a GI score of 42) with fruit and yoghurt is converted by the body into energy at a much slower rate. This type of breakfast will provide us with a slow-releasing source of energy so that we can go about all of our morning activities without feeling hungry. We're not likely to want to eat again until lunchtime, when our blood sugar levels start to get a bit low.

Carbohydrates with a high GI score can be converted into fat tissue, which will make weight loss difficult. This is due to a fast rise followed by a fall in blood sugar levels. On the other hand, low-GI foods are converted slowly, keeping blood sugar levels balanced, which means that there is less need for the body to convert these foods into fat tissue. Therefore, a low-GI diet helps the body to shed excess weight better than a high GI diet *even if the exact same amount of calories are consumed.*

weight loss without struggle

So, the easiest way to reach your weight-loss goals is to make sure all the carbohydrates you eat have a low-to-moderate glycaemic index score. This strategy will help you avoid hunger pangs and cravings and create the ideal conditions for your metabolism to burn off excess weight easily and permanently. The table below provides the GI values of different foods. In general, refined foods have a higher GI than unrefined, so choose brown rice and wholegrain bread over white rice and white bread. Unrefined foods contain a much higher level of nutrients as well.

Fruit makes an ideal snack if you feel peckish between meals as it usually has a low GI. Nuts and seeds are also low-GI foods. Combining low-to-moderate GI foods with a little protein or fat also helps to slow down the rate at which they are converted to energy, which keeps us feeling full for longer. For example, adding flax seeds and a couple of tablespoons of soya yoghurt to muesli or porridge would reduce the energy conversion of this meal even further and keep you feeling full of energy and alert throughout the morning.

A few foods that have a high GI can still form part of your diet, as they are healthy in all other respects. Baked potatoes can be eaten with beans or a protein food such as tuna, which will slow down the conversion substantially. Although watermelon has a high GI, the actual energy content is quite low so it won't unbalance your blood sugar levels.

It is important to eat regularly to keep your metabolic rate working properly so that you can lose weight without struggle and keep it off permanently. Try to eat breakfast, as your blood sugar is naturally low when you wake up. *Breakfast will kick-start your metabolic rate into action, so even if you don't like to eat immediately upon rising, try to have something within an hour or so.* Most of the popular breakfast cereals have a high GI so these should be avoided in favour of porridge, buckwheat flakes or a good-quality muesli purchased from the health-food shop.

glycaemic index of different foods[1]

low-GI foods	moderate-GI foods	high-GI foods
Kidney beans 28	Rice, brown 50	Rice, white 69
Lentils 29	Pitta bread 57	White bread 73
Chickpeas 28	Sweetcorn 46	French fries 75
Butter beans 31	New potatoes,	Potato, baked 85
Houmous 10	boiled 50	Popcorn 72
Soya beans 18	Baked beans,	Pretzels 83
Porridge,	sugar 48	Cornflakes 81
whole oats 42	Spaghetti 57	French baguette 95
Barley kernel	Muesli 49	Puffed rice 87
bread[1] 34	Wholemeal rye	Gluten-free bread 76
Pearl barley 25	bread 58	Weetabix 75
Cashew nuts 22	Oat bran bread[2] 47	Rice cakes 78
Yoghurt 30	Buckwheat 54	Bagels 72
Soya milk 40	Rye crispbread 64	Pumpkin 75
Soya fruit smoothie 30	Wholewheat	Lucozade 95
Yam 37	bread 52	Puffed wheat 80
Apricots, dried 31	Peas, green 48	Shredded Wheat 83
Apples 38	Carrot juice 43	Lychees, canned 78
Apple juice 40	Banana 52	Corn chips 72
Grapefruit 25	Orange juice,	Watermelon 72
Carrots, boiled 32	no sugar 52	Doughnuts 76
Cherries 22	Mango 51	Parsnips 97
Pears 38	Figs, dried 61	Sports drinks 70+
Oranges 42	Pineapple 59	Maltose 100
Peaches, fresh 42	Papaya 56	
Fructose (fruit sugar) 20	Grapes 46	
	Apricots (fresh) 57	
	Honey 55	

[1] 80% whole barley kernels
[2] 50% oat bran

As you can see, the eating plan you have been following on the Dairy-free Detox Diet has also been emphasizing low-GI rather than high-GI foods. In fact, eating a diet based on low-to-moderate GI foods should become a way of life, even after you have achieved your ideal weight. These foods are also packed with nutrients and contain lots of soluble fibre that will help the digestive system.

There are lots of other factors of this diet that will assist your efforts to lose weight. These include eating an alkaline-forming diet and adding small amounts of essential fats to your diet each day. The essential fats help to keep your metabolism working at its best, while a highly alkaline-forming diet helps to create the right biochemical conditions for the body to shed both excess fluid and fat tissue. Eating a nutritious diet, such as you are doing here, also helps to keep food cravings at bay.

Most people notice such a significant improvement to their overall wellbeing when switching to a low-GI diet that it's easy to make this a normal way of eating. These include an increase in energy levels, more balanced emotions and a clearer mind. As mentioned, premenstrual symptoms such as cravings for sugary foods and depression usually clear up within a short while of eating a diet based on low-GI foods. Other health benefits associated with eating plenty of low-to-moderate GI foods and avoiding high GI foods include a reduced risk of diabetes, heart disease and cancer.[2]

overcoming comfort eating

Avoiding intolerant foods and eating a diet with plenty of low-GI foods will greatly reduce any problems you may have with cravings and support your metabolism. Food cravings that are psychological in nature, however, are obviously different to physical cravings. **We all succumb to psychological food cravings from time to time. Who has never reached for a chocolate bar after a hard day? This behaviour is natural, as we have been 'programmed' to associate food with nurturing and comfort since early childhood.**

use positive alternatives

This pattern can become such an ingrained habit, though, that we turn to food each and every time we feel stressed or upset, or even when we have something to celebrate. Trying to break this pattern with willpower alone can be very hard. A better approach is to have a range of alternative activities that will stop us using food as a form of emotional support. We can usually get hold of a piece of chocolate cake or packet of crisps (chips) within a few minutes, so the alternative activities we choose to break this habit also have to be fast and easy to do or they won't work.

If you know that comfort eating has been hampering your efforts to lose weight, spend a few minutes developing substitute activities that will help you to break this pattern. For example, a friend of mine always carries a small bottle of lemon essential oil in her bag. She reaches for this and takes a whiff once in a while when she notices she's feeling a bit pressured or down. The smell reminds her of a place in Italy she visits frequently and would one day like to live. This small action, which takes only a few seconds, always makes her feel good. Other ideas along the same lines are:

- Making a quick call to a supportive friend.
- Taking a short walk, paying particular attention to things you find beautiful.
- Taking a minute or two to connect with your breathing while thinking about things that are good in your life right now.
- Doing something physical, such as standing up and having a good stretch and shake. Moving your body gets your energy flowing again and usually helps to improve your mood as well.

treat yourself

Another approach is to reward yourself with a treat for resisting the urge to comfort-eat. Lots of little treats rather than one more distant goal generally work best. For example:

- a new CD
- a long soak in the bath
- a manicure
- a bunch of flowers
- a home facial

This will soon start to create a self-enforcing pattern and you will feel really good about yourself.

Listen to Your Feelings

It also helps to spend some time exploring what your emotions are trying to tell you. Comfort eating may be a signal that an area of your life isn't working as well as you would like. So rather than ignoring the message, listen to what your inner guidance is saying and, if appropriate, make some changes to your life.

listening to your body

If you have been a yo-yo dieter, or you have had a strong tendency towards food cravings (either physical or psychological), you may well have lost touch with your body's signals for both hunger and feeling full. A low-GI diet really helps to reconnect to these natural signals. Working with them will make achieving your ideal weight much easier.

A good strategy is to eat only when you have a genuine physical feeling of hunger. This physical sensation can be described as feeling 'pleasantly peckish'. Ignoring this body signal for any length of time will result in your blood sugar levels falling too low, making it more likely that you will overeat later. If you're feeling a bit peckish but know you're having a meal within an hour or so, have a small snack such as fruit, a handful of nuts or rye crispbread with houmous.

If there is no tangible physical sensation associated with your desire to eat, this is probably either an emotional signal urging you to comfort-eat or simply a desire to eat for the enjoyment of it. So, take a moment before you eat to ask yourself 'Am I genuinely hungry?', and tune in to your emotions to find out how you are feeling.

It usually takes 10–15 minutes for the stomach to tell the brain that it is full. Eating slowly will help you notice the physical sensations of getting full. Don't put too large a portion of food on your plate, as there will be the temptation to eat it all, even if you are full. You can always go back for another portion later if you still feel hungry. Don't eat beyond the feeling of comfortable fullness.

summary

Eating low-to-moderate GI foods, along with a balanced diet containing protein and some essential fats, while following your body's signals for hunger and satiation is a highly effective strategy for achieving permanent weight loss. It's also important to avoid empty calories, such as sugary processed foods (which are high-GI foods anyway), saturated fat and alcohol. Finally, make sure you drink plenty of water. Apart from the other health benefits, it's easy to confuse the body's request for water with a signal for hunger. Try to exercise at least three times a week as this will help keep your metabolism functioning at its best. It will also protect your bones and your overall health.

To sum up, here are the main strategies to help you reach your ideal weight and keep it there in the long term:

- Eat three meals a day, with carbohydrate sources being mainly low- or moderate-GI foods.
- Combine a small amount of protein foods with carbohydrates so that they are released even more slowly.
- A small amount of essential fats in your diet will help you lose weight and support your overall health.

- Eat plenty of alkaline-forming foods.
- Drink plenty of water so that you don't confuse thirst with hunger. Don't drink too much with meals.
- Only eat when you are genuinely hungry. Eat when you have the physical sensation of being 'pleasantly peckish' but don't allow yourself to get hungrier than this.
- Try not to skip meals, especially breakfast.
- Keep your portion sizes modest. You can always go back for second helpings.
- Eat slowly and stop eating before you feel completely full.
- Have substitute activities to break the pattern of comfort eating.
- Avoid empty calories.
- Exercise regularly.

13: calcium and other important nutrients

It's a myth that we have to eat dairy foods to get enough calcium in our diet, as lots of other foods contain this mineral. We usually think of calcium in terms of strong bones, but it also plays a role in many other important functions, including:

- maintaining proper nerve impulses and muscle contractions
- regulating the heartbeat
- blood clotting
- detoxifying heavy metals such as lead

This chapter shows you how to get sufficient calcium in your diet and, importantly, how to balance your calcium intake with other essential nutrients such as magnesium.

calcium requirements

The recommended intake of calcium for adults in the UK is 800mg per day; in the US it is 1,000mg. Women who are breast-feeding need about 500mg more than this. Our need for calcium varies from person to person, depending on our diet and lifestyle habits. For example, if our diet is high in protein and we take lots of exercise, we will need more calcium than the average person. In general, an intake of 800–1,000mg per day should be ample for most people's needs.

When it comes to nutrition, it's certainly not the case that more is better. As mentioned earlier, too much calcium can lead to the calcification, or hardening, of soft body tissue such as the muscles, heart and kidneys. It may also increase the risk of prostate cancer. Moreover, high doses of calcium *on its own* appear to have at most a marginal (and sometimes detrimental) effect on bone health if the other nutrients that work alongside it are not considered.[1] Taking high quantities of calcium also increases the risk of developing deficiencies of other minerals. Key nutrients that need to be balanced with calcium are magnesium, vitamin D, vitamin B6 and vitamin K.

dietary sources of calcium

Lots of foods contain good quantities of calcium so, with care and attention, it isn't difficult to get your daily intake without eating dairy. Fish such as sardines, whitebait and salmon provide a valuable source of calcium (the calcium is in the edible bones). One medium-sized serving (115g/4oz) of sardines provides over 400mg of calcium. Nuts and seeds are also high-calcium foods, as are soya products. Sesame seeds, which are particularly high in calcium, also provide a rich source of the antioxidant mineral selenium (which is often deficient in the diet) and the omega-3 and omega-6 essential fats. Most leafy green vegetables contain moderate amounts of calcium but you do need to eat quite a lot of them to get an adequate intake. Although spinach is high in calcium, it is not a good source as we can absorb only a very tiny fraction of it.

good sources of calcium

Chinese vegetables	Hazelnuts
Sesame seeds (unhulled)	Figs (dried and fresh)
Tahini (ground sesame paste)	Broccoli
Sardines, with edible bones	Watercress
Salmon, with edible bones	Sunflower seeds
Whitebait, sprats	Parsley
Trout	Other herbs
Almonds	

calcium-enriched foods

Calcium-enriched soya milk	Calcium-enriched rice milk
Calcium-enriched tofu	Calcium-enriched orange juice*

* Available in North America but not in the UK

We can easily boost our calcium intake by buying products that have added calcium, such as fortified rice milk, soya milk and tofu. Some cereals are enriched with calcium, but given that these products often contain high levels of salt and sugar, they should be consumed sparingly.

Here are two sample menus that illustrate how easy it is for you to get enough calcium in your daily diet. For a full list of the calcium content of different foods, *see Appendix 4.*

sample menus providing plenty of calcium

non-vegetarian	calcium	vegetarian/vegan	calcium
BREAKFAST		BREAKFAST	
Boiled egg, toast, honey	30mg	Toast with almond butter	83 mg
Freshly squeezed orange		Fruit salad with soya	
juice	27mg	yoghurt and sesame	
Cereal with fortified rice		seeds:	
milk	240mg	Fruit, mixed	25mg
		Soya yoghurt, 3oz	125mg
		Sesame seeds, ¼oz	72mg
		Fresh squeezed	20mg
		grapefruit juice	
LUNCH		LUNCH	
Sardines, baked potato with tahini,		Falafel, houmous, pitta bread	
and salad:		with a watercress salad:	
Sardines, 4oz	413mg	Falafel, 3oz	40 mg
Potato	20mg	Houmous, 1oz	58mg
Tahini, 2 tbsp	128mg	Pitta bread	neg
Lettuce, tomato,		Watercress, 2oz	80mg
avocado	12mg	Tomato, cucumber	10mg
Olive oil dressing	neg.		
Fruit salad	25mg		
DINNER		DINNER	
Chicken, pasta with broccoli		Stir-fry tofu and vegetables with	
and okra:		rice:	
Chicken, pasta	neg.	Fortified tofu, 4oz	258mg
Broccoli 3oz	50mg	Broccoli, 2oz	34mg
Okra 3oz	63mg	Chinese cabbage, 1oz	106mg
		Other vegetables	10mg
		Rice	neg.
SNACKS		SNACKS	
1 banana	8mg	3 figs (dried or fresh)	81mg
1 apple	10mg	Pistachio nuts, 1 oz	40mg
1 grapefruit	30mg	1 apple	10mg
Estimated total calcium intake: 1,056 mg		Estimated total calcium intake: 1,052 mg	

magnificent magnesium

Vitamins and minerals never work in isolation – they work with other nutrients in teams. **Magnesium is the twin sister of calcium. These two minerals work closely together in maintaining many vital bodily functions.** For example, both calcium and magnesium are needed in a balanced ratio to keep your heart pumping properly – calcium provides the stimulus for your heart to contract while magnesium prompts the heart to relax. Exactly the same role is performed by these nutrients to move and relax your muscles. A balanced ratio between calcium and magnesium also ensures that blood clotting is kept within a healthy range; if calcium is not balanced with sufficient magnesium, there is a risk of thrombosis.[2] Magnesium also plays a crucial role in literally hundreds of enzyme functions including regulating blood pressure, balancing blood sugar and preventing kidney stones.

A healthy balance between calcium and magnesium is in the region of 3:2 in favour of calcium. Although dairy products do contain some magnesium, there is 11mg of calcium for 1mg of magnesium. A high consumption of dairy products increases the risk of magnesium deficiency because large intakes of calcium decrease magnesium absorption.[3]

Did You Know?

Magnesium deficiency is very common. The recommended intake of magnesium in the UK is 300mg for men and 270mg for women but many people fall short of this amount. Magnesium deficiency is associated with symptoms such as muscle cramps, insomnia, high blood pressure, fatigue, unstable blood sugar levels, PMS, menstrual pains and heart attacks.

Magnesium is just as important as calcium for keeping our bones healthy. In fact, some scientists believe that osteoporosis is actually a symptom of magnesium, rather than calcium, deficiency.[4] Magnesium has a number of functions to play in keeping our bones healthy:

- It assists with calcium absorption.
- It is essential for maintaining the health of the parathyroid gland (hormones from this gland influence bone strength).
- It is necessary for the proper metabolism of both vitamin D and calcium.[5]
- It forms part of the bone structure.
- It directly stimulates the cells that build bone.[6]

Several research studies have found that women with osteoporosis are deficient in magnesium.[7,8] Increasing magnesium intake over a period of two years has reduced fractures and improved bone density.[9,10]

Given that magnesium is so valuable to our health, we should aim to eat some high-magnesium foods every day. The table below lists some of the best dietary sources of magnesium. Most of these foods are also high in calcium and, unlike dairy products, provide a balanced ratio of both minerals. Sugar is an enemy of magnesium as it promotes loss of this mineral via the kidneys, so this is another reason to keep your intake of sugary foods low.

sources of magnesium

Pumpkin seeds	Okra
Sunflower seeds	Figs
Sesame seeds	Sprouted seeds/beans (alfalfa, mung)
Almonds	Broccoli
Hazelnuts	Beetroot
Brazil nuts	Wheat germ
Shrimp	Lima beans
Tofu	Brown rice (not white)

other important nutrients

vitamin D

Calcium absorption is enhanced with the presence of vitamin D. This vitamin is also involved with maintaining the balance of calcium in blood and bone. We don't need much vitamin D. An intake of 400iu per day is usually sufficient. If we live in sunny climes, we can easily produce all that we need from the action of sunlight on our skin. Dietary sources of vitamin D are shown below. As it is stored in the liver, it is not necessary to eat foods containing this vitamin every day. In fact, excess levels of vitamin D can be toxic resulting in nausea, constant thirst and headaches. Although it is unlikely that someone can take in excessive amounts from diet alone, this is a real possibility when taking large amounts of fish liver oil supplements, which are high in both vitamin D and vitamin A (omega-3 fish oil supplements do not contain vitamins A and D).

vitamin K

This is another important bone-enhancing nutrient that helps the body maintain calcium balance and inhibits bone breakdown. A group of Harvard researchers monitored the dietary habits of over 72,000 women over a period of 10 years. After taking account of other bone health factors (such as calcium and protein intake), women who had a high vitamin K intake had a significantly reduced rate of hip fractures than those whose intake was low. Lettuce on its own (a good source of vitamin K) reduced fracture risk by 45 per cent for women who consumed it at least once a day compared with women who ate lettuce a couple of times a week.[11]

potassium

This mineral, found in abundance in fruits and vegetables, also helps to promote bone health.

sources of vitamin D and vitamin K

vitamin D	vitamin K
Herring	Cruciferous vegetables (cauliflower,
Mackerel	Brussels sprouts, cabbage, broccoli)
Salmon	Lettuce
Eggs	Potatoes
Wheat germ	Watercress
Fish liver oil supplements	Tomatoes
Sunlight	Peas (green)

Following the eating plan outlined in earlier chapters should ensure that you are getting plenty of vitamin K in your diet. The friendly bacteria that reside in the digestive tract also help the body to produce its own vitamin K. Here are a few simple ways of making sure you are getting plenty of calcium, magnesium and vitamins D and K in your diet.

- Sprinkle sesame seeds into soups, salads and breakfast cereals.
- Have a small handful of mixed nuts and seeds each day.
- Always have a portion of green vegetables or a salad with lunch and dinner.
- Eat sardines, salmon or mackerel at least three times a week.
- Eat tofu or soya yoghurt at least three times a week.
- Use small amounts of tahini or nut butter on toast instead of butter or jam.
- Use plenty of fresh herbs in salads, soups and stir-fries as they usually have a high mineral content (e.g. parsley, coriander and basil).
- Choose unprocessed foods (brown rice, wholemeal bread) instead of processed foods (white rice, white bread) as the nutrient content will be higher.
- Weather permitting, have a small amount of sun exposure each day. Remember to protect your skin from sun damage.
- Vary the foods you choose so that you are getting a wide mix of all these valuable nutrients.

- If your calcium requirements are particularly high (such as if you are breast-feeding) or if you don't eat foods naturally high in calcium, use calcium-fortified soya and rice milks on breakfast cereals, in smoothies and in cooking.

As you can see, these recommendations support other suggestions given elsewhere in this book. Following these guidelines also provides plenty of omega essential fats. These suggestions also provide low-to-moderate GI foods and alkaline-forming foods.

supplements

By far the best approach is to meet our nutrient requirements directly from food. But if you believe you can't get all you need from food then you may choose to supplement. There are several different forms of calcium supplement on the market. The ones to look out for are calcium citrate, chelated calcium or calcium carbonate. Food-form calcium, which is manufactured as close to food as possible, is also excellent. Avoid bonemeal and dolomite supplements as they are not easily absorbed and can contain high levels of lead, which is highly toxic.

Unless you've been advised to do so by a nutritionist or nutritionally-minded doctor, it isn't a good idea to take a calcium supplement on its own. Instead, balance calcium with sufficient magnesium, usually in a ratio of 3:2. Therefore, a good combination would be 300mg of calcium with 200mg of magnesium (with the remainder derived from diet). This is normally met by a good quality multimineral supplement.

If you are deficient in magnesium, the ratio would change to boost magnesium, such as 300mg of calcium with 300mg of magnesium (or you might supplement magnesium on its own for a couple of months). Good forms of magnesium are citrate, chelated magnesium or food form. If you take too high a dose of magnesium, you may get diarrhoea. Don't take a vitamin C supplement at the same time as your mineral supplement as they do not react well together. As mentioned earlier,

the best time to take your mineral supplement is just before going to bed as it will help to relax you and promote deep and restful sleep.

We need enough vitamin B6 in our diet for magnesium to do its job properly. Good sources of vitamin B6 include:

- nuts
- seeds
- lentils
- bananas
- kidney beans
- avocado
- meat

This chapter has shown you that it is relatively easy to meet your calcium requirements without resorting to dairy products. More importantly, it is the balance between calcium and other vital nutrients such as magnesium that is the key to achieving optimum health and well-being, including healthy bones. The next chapter discusses other important dietary and lifestyle factors that impact bone health.

14: beyond calcium – how to look after your bones

For healthy bones, you need calcium in balance with other nutrients such as magnesium, vitamins K and D and potassium, as we have seen. But to keep your bones healthy, you also need to make sure that your diet and lifestyle do not cause too much calcium and other minerals to be lost from your body. This is just as important – if not more so – as making sure your diet supplies calcium and related nutrients.[1]

osteoporosis

Osteoporosis, which literally means 'porous bones', is a severely crippling disease. It doesn't just affect elderly women; **it's estimated that many women in their 30s and 40s are already suffering from reduced bone mass.** And while the rates of osteoporosis are higher for women, men are by no means immune. It is often called the 'silent disease' because there are no symptoms (i.e. fractures) until bone loss has become extensive.

The number of people suffering with osteoporosis is steadily increasing; in fact, the World Health Organization is predicting an osteoporosis epidemic within the next few decades.[2] Therefore, it makes good sense to follow a few simple dietary and lifestyle strategies that can prevent or reduce the likelihood of you suffering with this disease. The younger you are when you start to look after your bones the better. But you will still benefit from these strategies even if you are older.

balancing the mineral bank account

The majority (99 per cent) of the calcium in the body resides in bones with the remaining 1 per cent circulating in blood and bodily fluids. Your bones act as an instant-access deposit account that the body draws from whenever it needs extra calcium and other mineral supplies. If your mineral 'income' (dietary intake) is less than what the body 'spends' (what your body uses), you will have a negative calcium balance – your body is essentially reducing its bone mass in order to meet current requirements.

In the same way that spending more than you earn will eventually lead to severe financial problems, so consistently having a negative calcium balance will eventually result in declining bone health. While the last chapter looked at ways of getting minerals and related nutrients in your diet, this chapter outlines ways in which you can cut back on unnecessary 'spending' of calcium so that you do not suffer with a negative calcium balance.

acid–alkaline balance

As you've already seen in earlier chapters, the overall acid–alkaline balance in the diet contributes significantly to calcium balance. Too many acid-forming foods (proteins and grains) and a lack of alkaline-forming foods are likely to result in a negative calcium balance – calcium is taken from bone to metabolize acid-ash waste products. A vast body of scientific research has found that a very high-protein diet, if not balanced with plenty of alkaline-forming foods, can negatively affect bone health.[3] There is also evidence that excess protein can have a direct detrimental effect on the cells responsible for bone breakdown and regeneration.[4]

On the other hand, a diet containing lots of alkaline-forming fruits and vegetables provides plenty of nutrients that improve calcium balance and protect your bones. These include magnesium and potassium, but also antioxidants such as vitamin C and betacarotene, which may reduce the risk of free-radical damage to the bone structure itself.[5]

When a group of scientists monitored the eating habits of an elderly group of men and women over four years, they found that those who regularly consumed lots of fruits and vegetables had less bone loss than those who had lower intakes of these foods. They summed up these findings by stating *'alkaline-producing dietary components, specifically, potassium, magnesium, and fruit and vegetables, contribute to maintenance of bone mineral density'.*[6]

The eating plan you have been following on the Dairy-free Detox Diet is therefore bone-healthy. Remember that protein foods play an important role in maintaining our health; we just need to make sure that the overall acid–alkaline components of our diet are in balance. An imbalance of acid-to-alkaline foods is the main dietary contributor to negative mineral balance. Here are other nutritional and lifestyle factors that do the same thing.

salt

Table salt (sodium chloride) has a significant negative impact on calcium balance. It has been estimated that just one extra gram of salt per day would, if dealt with totally from the calcium in bones, reduce bone mass by 1 per cent per year.[7] It's actually the chloride molecules in table salt that produce the excretion of calcium.[8] Natural salts (organic sodium) are found in most fruits and vegetables and these don't have a negative impact on calcium balance.

oxalates and phytates

These substances are part of the indigestible fibre in certain foods. The minerals in your diet bind with them and pass unabsorbed through the digestive tract. Spinach and rhubarb have very high oxalate levels. They are otherwise healthy foods but try to eat them sparingly. A portion of boiled spinach contains approximately 244mg of calcium but only 5mg of calcium will actually be absorbed by the body. Other foods that contain moderate amounts of oxalates include celery, chocolate, tea and green beans.

Phytates are mainly found in grains, particularly wheat. Wheat bran is also very high in oxalates. In other words, wheat bran can significantly decrease mineral absorption leading to deficiencies in calcium, magnesium and zinc. Soya has a high phytate content but is exceptional in that the calcium content is nevertheless still well absorbed. Soya foods also encourage the body to store calcium. A high-fibre diet derived from fruit and vegetables (which consist of soluble fibre rather than phytates) does not result in a negative calcium balance.[9] In fact, a diet high in soluble fibre enhances mineral absorption.[10]

alcohol

There is some evidence to suggest that moderate amounts of alcohol (one drink per day) may have a small protective effect on bone health in post-menopausal women.[11] This is because modest levels of alcohol can help the body produce small amounts of oestrogen. However, greater intakes of alcohol have been found to affect calcium absorption negatively so it's advisable to keep alcohol intake low.[12]

cola drinks and caffeine

Cola drinks contain phosphoric acid, which is highly acidic and causes quite a large amount of calcium to be lost in the urine.[13] Caffeine can also have a modest negative effect on calcium balance so it's best to keep coffee and tea intake low.

lifestyle factors

Certain lifestyle factors can have a positive or negative impact on our bones.

exercise

Regular weight-bearing exercise, such as gentle jogging or stair climbing, is one of the best things you can do to keep your bones healthy. Swimming, although excellent for your heart and overall fitness levels, isn't the best exercise for promoting bone strength. The buoyancy of the water means there is virtually no weight-bearing impact on your bones. Weight-lifting is excellent. Three sessions of 20 minutes per week is sufficient and will tone (rather than build) your muscles as well. If you have never done weight-training before, work with a fitness trainer for a while who can show you how to use the weights properly. Activities such as yoga and t'ai chi are also fantastic as they help us develop a good sense of balance, which reduces the risk of us falling when we are older.

smoking

Smoking is extremely detrimental to bone health. It's been estimated that a woman who smokes one pack of cigarettes per day during her adult life would have a 10 per cent decline in bone density by the time she reaches menopause.[14] So this is yet another reason to avoid cigarettes.

depression and stress

Finally, depression and stress can weaken bone density.[15] This is because the hormones that are released when we experience these emotions deplete calcium balance and directly suppress the activity of the cells responsible for rebuilding bone. We are only just beginning to understand the full effect our emotions have on our physical health. But looking after our emotions will help us to protect our bones and overall health as well.

15: side-effects of modern dairy farming

Dairy farming traditionally consisted of lots of small farms that would supply their local community with milk, butter and cheese. But those days are long gone. The poor profitability of dairy farming – the farmer only receives one third from the retail price of a pint of milk – has resulted in many small farms simply being unable to survive. And the larger farms (the average herd size in the United States is 9,000) have been keen to devise strategies that will increase the amount of milk a cow can produce.

In this respect, farmers have been quite successful, as **the average milk yield per cow has doubled during the past 20 years. But this success has not been without a cost, both in terms of animal welfare and the potential negative impact on human health.** Cows now produce up to 20 times more milk per year than is needed to suckle their calves. Furthermore, cows are made to give birth every year, which means that they continue to be milked during the period that they are pregnant. This increase in milk production could not have been achieved if cows were left to graze in open pastures; rather, farmers now add high-protein dry feeds to the cows' diets. Although the lifespan of cows is more than a dozen years, they are frequently culled at the age of three.

I don't believe that dairy farmers are evil sadists hell-bent on torturing the animals in their care. I'm sure that most are decent, hard-working and caring individuals simply attempting to make a living for themselves and their families. But the use of certain farming practices, in particular the large-scale use of antibiotics and hormones to increase growth and milk yields, are highly questionable both in terms of animal welfare and in the wider perspective of human and environmental health.

antibiotics and the superbug issue

Modern farming methods have not been without their negative consequences. Mastitis, a very painful udder infection, is a common disease among dairy cows. Lameness also affects about 25 per cent of cows each year due to problems associated with excessively large udders, poor housing and high-protein diets. The usual treatment for these conditions is antibiotics, principally the beta-lactan penicillins.

However, cows are also regularly given antibiotic injections purely for growth-promoting purposes, as this drug makes the cow produce more milk. Further, these drugs are frequently mixed into the cows' food in order to destroy any micro-organisms that may reside in the high-protein dry mix. Finally, as a purely preventative measure against mastitis, antibiotics are given to cows via tubes inserted into their udders. Although there are strict government regulations and regular screening to ensure that antibiotics do not make their way into our milk supply, trace amounts of the drug can seep through. This means that we are getting unnecessary exposure to antibiotics, which can result in all sorts of health problems.

Antibiotics, which literally mean 'against life', were designed to kill bacteria. When antibiotics were first developed, they were heralded as the ultimate cure for a number of life-threatening diseases. But what scientists didn't anticipate was the tenacity and resilience of bacteria to being eradicated. Bacteria have lived on this planet for billions of years and during this time they've learned a thing or two about survival. Bacteria have the ability to transform and mutate so that they very quickly become resistant to a particular antibiotic drug. During the past few decades there has been an on-going race between the antibiotic manufacturers and bacteria. A new antibiotic is effective for a while, but as the bacteria quickly mutate, the drug no longer has an effect. This forces the drug manufacturers to make another, stronger antibiotic. But yet again the bacteria simply mutate and build resistance to the new drug.

In terms of winning the race, the bacteria are outwitting the scientists hands down. If there were an infinite number of new antibiotics, the rapid development of bacterial resistance wouldn't be a problem. But we are running out of new antibiotics very fast. So although we've had 50 years or so of remission from bacteria-provoked disease, we're on the threshold of releasing completely antibiotic-resistant strains of bacteria (the so-called superbugs) into the environment. We are already seeing the beginnings of this problem with superbugs such as MRSA being commonplace in many hospitals.

About 750 tonnes of antibiotics are used in animal farming in the UK each year. This is approximately 50 per cent more than that used for humans (560 tonnes per year). However, the vast majority of antibiotic use in farming is totally unnecessary as the drugs are used solely to support unhealthy intensive farming practices. One third, or 250 tonnes, of the antibiotics used in animal farming are there solely for growth-promoting purposes.[1] But the short-term gain for the farmer is increasing the risk of long-term havoc that will occur if the superbug problem accelerates. **The antibiotics used in farming are the same as those used to treat human health problems, meaning that bacterial resistance can easily spread across species.** The World Health Organization states that antibiotic-resistant strains of bacteria such as salmonella and E. coli have already been transmitted from animals to humans.

Dairy farming is not the only industry that uses lots of antibiotics. Unfortunately, the problem is endemic throughout animal farming. We also expose ourselves to antibiotic residues every time we eat meat, particularly chicken. As consumers, we can make our voice heard by voting with our wallets and choosing organic products where antibiotics are only used when absolutely necessary.

sneaking in genetically-modified organisms

Many dairy farmers in the United States use a genetically-modified growth hormone to boost milk yields. This hormone, rBST (also known as rBGH and with the trade name *Posilac*), which is produced by Monsanto and other biotechnology firms, mimics the cow's own hormone, insulin-growth factor-1 (IGF-1). Injecting cows with rBST increases milk yield by 10–15 per cent. The Food and Drug Administration in the United States has allowed this drug to be used since the early 1990s and claims that it poses no threat to humans. However, it is banned in many other countries around the world.

Humans also produce IGF-1, which is essential for the proper development during childhood and adolescence of breast tissue and the prostate gland. However, too much IGF-1 during adulthood is known to be a potent risk factor for the development of cancers of the breast and prostate (as it causes cancer cell growth). The milk of cows treated with rBST contains 10 times more IGF-1 than the milk of untreated cows. IGF-1 in cow's milk is molecularly virtually identical to the human hormone, suggesting that these dairy products could pose a serious health threat to humans. Exposure to IGF-1 is also believed to be a risk factor in other serious health conditions such as infertility, birth defects and damage to the immune system.

Ben and Jerry's Ice Cream is one of the few American firms that have made a public declaration that they will not use rBST milk in their products. But in general it is impossible to know whether a particular pint of milk (or other dairy product) was derived from rBST-treated cows, as milk from different farms is mixed together before reaching the supermarket shelves. The only way to be sure is to buy organic dairy products, which are definitely rBST-free.

Because of the very serious health concerns over the use of rBST, it has been banned in Canada, Europe, Australia, New Zealand and Japan. However, there is no legal restraint in the UK against selling imported products that contain dairy products derived from cows treated with this hormone. There are lots of American dairy products available in the UK such as pizza, ice cream and cheese. Unless you are in the minority that believes rBST won't damage your health, it's best to avoid these products.

There is also the important issue of animal welfare, as cows treated with rBST have increased incidence of mastitis and other diseases. Again, this means that yet more antibiotics need to be given to the cow.

This is not only bad for the animals but also a further unnecessary threat that antibiotic-resistant bacteria will evolve.

Enzymes are required to make cheese curdle. The most common of these is rennet, which is derived from the inside of the stomach of dead calves. Vegetarian cheese normally contains plant-derived enzymes, but in some cases a genetically-engineered bacteria (chymosin) that mimics rennet is used. There is no legal requirement in the UK to put this information on the label, meaning that many consumers are unwittingly eating genetically-engineered cheese. The Co-Op is the only supermarket in the UK that voluntarily informs customers by stating on the label that GM chymosin has been used.[2]

hormone disrupters, pesticides and the cocktail effect

In their quest for greater milk yields, dairy farmers are permitted to give cows hormone treatments, including oestradiol (a form of oestrogen, similar to that used in hormone replacement therapy for post-menopausal women). Cows are regularly milked while they are pregnant (up to month seven of a nine-month gestation), a period when their natural oestrogen levels are high. Hormone residues can pass through into milk, where they can disrupt human hormone balance. Furthermore, there are 500 pesticides legally permitted for use on dairy farms.[3]

Environmental pollutants also have hormone-disrupting effects. These include PCBs, organo-chlorine chemicals such as DDT, and dioxins. These are all man-made toxins, usually by-products of industrial manufacturing, which have made their way into our food supply. These persistent organic pollutants biodegrade very slowly, meaning that they remain in the environment for several years. Our primary exposure to PCBs, DDT and dioxins is from the foods we eat. These contaminants are found in small amounts in many foods, but the highest concentrations are found in fatty foods, especially dairy products, meat, eggs and fish.

All of these chemical substances have a particular affinity with fat, which is the reason why there are higher quantities of them in foods that contain fat. In other words, when an animal (or human) is exposed to these compounds, they will attach themselves to fatty tissue where they are stored. And with respect to dairy, the compounds will find their way into the cow's milk, which also contains a high proportion of fat. Trace residues of dioxins and PCBs are regularly found in cow's milk.[4] Butter, which is 99 per cent fat, has also been found to contain these compounds as well as DDT. European butter typically has higher levels of DDT than butter produced in North America.[5] These residues have not been found in organic butter.[6]

In 1996, a government test found that 46 per cent of milk sampled contained the highly toxic pesticide lindane, with over 4 per cent containing amounts higher than the maximum safety level. Lindane residues have also been found in butter and cheese.[7] Lindane, which is a particularly toxic pesticide associated with nerve disorders and other serious diseases, has since been banned. But like other organo-chemicals, lindane compounds will remain in the environment for some time; hence small amounts can still make their way into our food supply. Humans are identical to animals when it comes to the way in which our bodies handle these chemical compounds. An assessment of human fatty tissue found traces of DDT in 99 per cent of the people sampled. Levels ranged from 1mg to 9mg per kilo of body weight, which are quite significant.[8] Similarly, PCBs, dioxins and DDT can all pass into human breast milk and hence be transferred to the infant.

All of these chemicals are believed to have several damaging consequences to health, which is why PCBs, lindane and DDT have been banned and dioxin emissions are severely restricted. The World Health Organization states that long-term exposure to these compounds is linked with hormone-related disorders, such as breast, prostate and testicular cancers, and infertility problems (male sperm counts have fallen dramatically over the past few decades). They are also associated with diseases of the nervous system and immune-related conditions.[9]

The problem with these contaminants is certainly not confined to dairy products. Levels of dioxins, PCBs and DDT are also regularly found in other foods. Because these pollutants have found their way into our oceans, fish can easily be contaminated. Two different batches of cod liver oil supplements had to be recalled during 2002 because they were found to contain high levels of PCBs.

The UK government has set maximum safety levels (TEQs) for the individual chemical compounds that are permitted in our food, and regular tests are conducted to make sure that limits are not exceeded. Amounts less than the maximum safety levels are deemed to be safe. But as substances like dioxins are damaging to health, it is certainly worth cutting down our exposure to even small amounts. The simplest way to do this is to reduce our intake of foods that contain high amounts of animal fat. Oily fish should be eaten only if you know it has come from relatively pollution-free waters. Check the labels on cod liver oil or fish oil supplements as the better quality products make sure that they are derived from pollution-free sources and will usually state this on this label. It's definitely worth paying that little bit extra for a contaminant-free product.

go organic

If, in the longer term, you choose to include some dairy products in your diet then it's best to go for organic products. Organic farmers let cows graze on pasture that has not been sprayed with pesticides; do not use growth hormones or any GM ingredients; and only give antibiotics to an animal if it is genuinely sick. This approach is infinitely preferable for the animal and provides dairy products that are better for our health.

The same recommendation goes for all the foods we eat. Fruits, vegetables and grains such as wheat are regularly treated with chemicals, and residues frequently remain on the foods. Although individual chemicals may be deemed safe in isolation, no research has considered the potentially damaging effects of the interactions that may occur from our long-term exposure to literally thousands of chemicals, the so-called 'cocktail effect'. Therefore it seems sensible to cut down our exposure as much as we can.

16: further information

This chapter contains further information on some of the processes described throughout the book. You don't need to read this chapter to follow the Dairy-free Detox Diet but many of you will want to know more about the science behind the dietary advice. Each heading gives the corresponding chapter number in brackets so you can refer to it if you like.

lactose intolerance and genes (chapter 2)

Dr Hollox and colleagues reported in the *American Journal of Human Genetics*[1] that they have found a specific genetic sequence that prompts lactase production to persist into adulthood. The only people who have this genetic sequence are of North European descent, where drinking animal milk has been relatively common for thousands of years. But even then it is estimated that only 30 per cent of North Europeans are able to produce lots of lactase in adulthood.[2] So although lactose intolerance is less frequent in Northern Europeans than in other ethnic groups, it is still quite common. To discover your chances of being lactose intolerant, see the following table.

percentage of people with lactase deficiency by ethnic region[3]

Asia (e.g. India, China, Japan)	90%
Africa	75%
MiddleEast	75%
Southern Europe (e.g. Spain, Greece)	75%
South America	75%
Native Americans	75%
Northern Europe	70%

the causes of food intolerance (chapter 3)

The following diagram shows how various factors, including lactose intolerance, can provoke a full-blown intolerance to dairy.

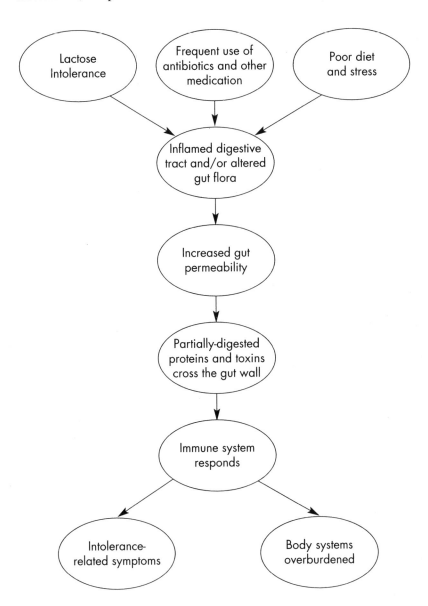

heart disease and dairy products (chapter 4)

Researchers have linked low-fat dairy products with an increased risk of cardiovascular disease. One explanation is the chemical compound homocysteine, which is now recognized to be a major factor that increases the risk of heart disease. Homocysteine is a highly toxic substance produced in the body after eating any type of protein. If there are plenty of B-vitamins in the diet (in particular B6, B12 and folic acid), this chemical is converted into a harmless form and excreted. But if B-vitamins are low then homocysteine can cause substantial damage to artery walls, resulting in cardiovascular disease. Some researchers have suggested that the level of homocysteine produced from drinking milk, which is a high-protein food, will be quite high. Milk contains even fewer B-vitamins than meat,[4] another high-protein food.

There is also some evidence that the lactose in milk and dairy products can be metabolized into fats that increase the levels of 'bad' cholesterol (VLDL).[5] This type of cholesterol is known to increase the risk of heart problems.

Calcium is an important nutrient, helping to maintain blood pressure within a normal range, but too much calcium in the diet – especially when it isn't balanced with other minerals – can cause problems. With respect to heart disease, excess calcium can result in calcification (hardening) of the arteries (arteriosclerosis), which can increase the likelihood of a heart attack or stroke. As was discussed in Chapter 3, the arachidonic acid found in dairy increases the stickiness of the blood, a further risk factor for cardiovascular problems.

the acid–alkaline balance (chapter 5)

When a cell is metabolizing nutrients, it acts like a miniature furnace that effectively 'burns' nutrients to release their intrinsic value. In the same way that ash remains after coals are burnt in the fire, so a metabolic ash remains in the cell after it has completed its work. This ash needs to be removed from the cell and eliminated from the body via the kidneys and intestines. The type of ash produced depends on the food that has been eaten. It doesn't matter whether the food is acid or alkaline in its natural state. A lemon is highly acidic but when it is metabolized it leaves an alkaline ash.

The body has developed buffering systems whose job is to neutralize any acid ash molecules. Once they are neutralized, they can be safely transported through the body into the elimination channels without causing any cellular damage. This is akin to how we would dispose of corrosive chemicals in our home. We don't just chuck them down the sink as this could cause damage to the pipes and the water supply. Instead we package or neutralize them in some way so that we can remove them without causing unnecessary harm.

The body's buffering systems require alkaline minerals, particularly sodium, calcium, magnesium and potassium. When the diet does not provide sufficient levels of these minerals, the body has no choice but to draw from the stock available in bones, which is primarily calcium. Thus, our bones act like a mineral bank account that can provide extra calcium for buffering support whenever it is needed. These minerals are subsequently eliminated in urine or faeces.

Note that it is organic sodium that is used in the buffering process (and many other bodily functions as well). Organic sodium is found in most fruits and vegetables. This form of sodium is completely different to table salt, which is sodium chloride. In fact, the chloride molecules in table salt have an acidifying effect on the body.

essential fatty acids (chapter 11)

When we munch on sunflower seeds or drizzle safflower oil onto our salad, we get a form of omega-6 called linoleic acid. Before the body can use linoleic acid, it has to undergo a three-step conversion (*see diagram*).

conversion pathway of essential fatty acids

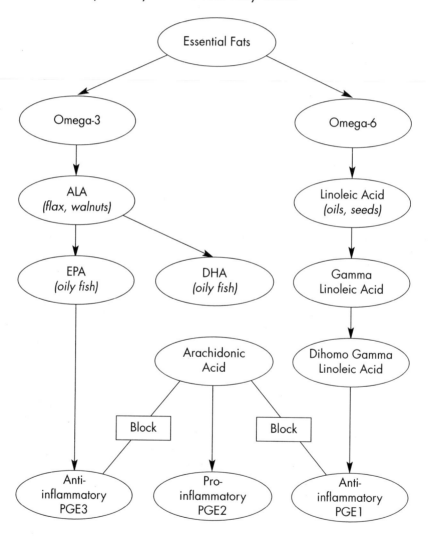

essential fatty acids and prostaglandins

Both omega-3 and the oils and seeds from the omega-6 family produce anti-inflammatory prostaglandins (PGE3 and PGE1 respectively). For example, it is the PGE3 produced from fish oils that is responsible for getting the body to reduce the stickiness of the blood. On the other hand, the arachidonic acid found in dairy foods and meat provokes a highly pro-inflammatory response (PGE2), which results in symptoms such as swelling, pain, rhinitis and increased blood thickness.

PMS symptoms such as period pains, heavy blood loss, food cravings and headaches can be associated with too much arachidonic acid, and hence an excess of PGE2. Other conditions associated with too much PGE2 include:

- rheumatoid arthritis
- migraines
- eczema
- hay fever
- asthma

The omega-6 seeds and oils that produce the anti-inflammatory PGE1 can help to alleviate all of these conditions. PGE1 also helps to balance blood sugar problems, which will reduce sugar cravings, mood swings and fatigue.

The body's ability to convert foods through all of the necessary stages to reach the end-product, prostaglandins, can be hampered by several factors. A diet high in dairy foods will promote an excessive amount of the inflammatory PGE2 and simultaneously block the ability to produce anti-inflammatory PGE1 and PGE3, even if sufficient good-quality foods containing these fats are consumed.

Eating a lot of saturated fat and/or trans fat in the diet will also block the prostaglandin conversion process while alcohol inhibits prostaglandin formation. The standard medical approach to inflammatory diseases such as eczema or rheumatoid arthritis is to prescribe non-steroid anti-inflammatory drugs. These will lead to an improvement in symptoms, as the levels of PGE2 will be reduced. But the drug also blocks the production of *all* prostaglandins, so they do not really provide a long-term solution.

Converting the omega-6 seeds and oils all the way through to PGE1 is quite a difficult process. Effective conversion depends upon a host of nutrients including vitamins B3, B6, biotin and C, plus magnesium and zinc, all of which are often low in the diet. Also, even if the correct nutrients are present, some people do not have sufficient levels of the specific enzymes (not digestive enzymes) to convert these foods properly.

If there is a family history of eczema, asthma or hay fever, it's likely there is a genetic deficiency of the enzymes needed for the conversion process. This means that even if the omega-6 fats are provided by the diet, the body will not be able to use them properly. A high intake of dairy foods can make these conditions worse as this will make it even harder for the body to produce PGE1.

GLA SUPPLEMENTS

Thankfully, there is a way around this problem, which you have already been following on the Dairy-free Detox Diet. The solution is to take nutritional supplements containing gamma linoleic acid (GLA), as this is already one step along the conversion process. GLA is also found in evening primrose or borage (starflower) oils.

Many people try evening primrose oil for a few months but find that it seems to have little effect. The reason is usually that the supplement did not contain a high enough dose of GLA to provide a therapeutic effect. A good supplementary dose of GLA is between 150–300mg per day, which is what you've been taking. Evening primrose oil contains approximately 10 per cent of this, so to get 150mg of GLA you need to take 1,500mg of evening primrose. Borage (starflower) oil contains about 15 per cent GLA.

Eczema usually responds well to GLA supplementation. In addition, you can open the GLA (or evening primrose) capsule and gently massage it directly onto sore skin. It has a very soothing and moisturizing effect. There is also evidence that omega-3 alleviates eczema problems, so the ideal strategy would be to take GLA and an omega-3 supplement simultaneously (or increase your intake of oily fish).[6] The same approach can be used if you suffer with PMS. Dry eyes, dry skin and dull hair also usually benefit from a GLA supplement. It's also important to reduce your intake of arachidonic acid, saturated fats and trans fats so that you give your body a chance to produce the healing PGE1 and PGE3 and avoid producing excess PGE2.

17: health for life

Several thousand years ago, Hippocrates, the founding father of Western medicine, said 'Let food be your medicine and medicine be your food'. This statement still holds true today. The rates of eczema, asthma, rheumatoid arthritis, diabetes and more serious illnesses such as heart disease, cancer, hormone-related problems and osteoporosis have been steadily increasing for several years. Yet it is widely accepted that diet and lifestyle influence all these health conditions, and many more. Health-care systems throughout the world are already overburdened. **We can help the overworked medical profession, and of course ourselves, by taking greater responsibility for our own health and wellbeing.** Making sure our diet is healthy is one of the most important ways in which we can do this.

Even though the relationship between diet and health has been known from Hippocratic times and earlier, nutritional science is still a relatively young field with new understandings emerging all the time. Nevertheless, we do currently have a pretty clear idea of the foods that harm and the foods that support our health. A diet high in processed foods packed with additives, saturated fat, trans fats, salt and sugar, caffeine-containing substances and alcohol will increase your risk of health problems. On the other hand, a diet consisting of whole foods such as fruits, vegetables, low-GI carbohydrates, good-quality protein foods and a small amount of essential fats will go a long way towards keeping us healthy throughout our lives. Eating organic where possible will take you that little bit further and will also help the environment.

As well as keeping us healthy, these foods also make us feel great. They give us lots of energy, keep our moods balanced and happy, and help the mind function at its best. **Healthy eating makes us look good, with clear skin, bright eyes, shiny hair, and a slim and vibrant body that doesn't suffer from bloating or puffiness.** You can achieve this type of diet whether you are a meat-eater (provided intake is kept low), fish-eater, vegetarian or vegan. The choice is yours, depending on your own tastes and beliefs.

Your body has a built-in wisdom that knows which foods to eat to maintain health. When our diet contains lots of sugar, salt, saturated fat and additives, or when we are suffering with a food intolerance problem, we may not hear these messages coming from the body as our whole system is overloaded. But as we make the switch to a healthier way of eating and address any food intolerance problems, we find that the body will tell us quite clearly which foods it needs at any particular time.

By combining your inner guidance with the knowledge you now have about the principles of a healthy diet, you can develop an eating plan that is perfect for your own needs. We are all constantly changing. At certain times we might feel a need for stimulation and outgoing activities, whereas at others we need more private and quiet time. Our nutritional needs will vary in the same way. One month we might find we have a taste for a few more protein foods. The next we may want to increase our intake of fruits and vegetables. This is both natural and healthy. Our eating pattern may also vary according to the influence of the seasons. Following your natural rhythms in this way can help you maintain a high level of health and wellbeing.

Of course, eating isn't just about keeping healthy. Food is one of life's great pleasures. With the health-promoting dietary principles described in this book, and Jane Sen's recipes, you can easily create a diet that is extremely tasty and delicious. Moreover, after you have been eating this way for a while, your taste in food will definitely change. Processed foods that are high in sugar, saturated fat and additives won't have the same appeal. But, as with most things in life, it's important to maintain balance. What you do day in, day out is what matters most. A piece of chocolate or a glass of champagne once in a while may be just what you need at that time and isn't going to damage your health. But eating lots of sugary foods or drinking a large amount of alcohol every day probably will.

Other factors such as looking after our emotions, having deep and meaningful relationships, creating work that reflects who we really are and regular exercise are also crucial for our overall health and wellbeing. But, as I hope you have experienced for yourself by following the suggestions in this book, overcoming a food intolerance problem and eating a nutritious, healthy diet can go a long way to keeping us feeling great, looking great and in good health for life.

Dawn Hamilton

18: the recipes

Ingredients are given for four servings per recipe.
Herbs and flavourings can be adjusted to suit individual tastes.
Oven temperatures for fan-assisted ovens should be adjusted according to manufacturer's instructions.

list of recipes

soups, salads and dressings

main dishes

puddings and cookies

soups, salads and dressings

egyptian-style chickpea, spinach and crispy pitta salad

2 wholewheat or white pitta breads	Split in half carefully, place in a hot oven and bake until crisp, taking care not to let them burn. Break into bite-size pieces and toss into a nice big bowl.

. . . .

200g/8oz/1½ cups cooked chickpeas (garbanzo beans) (use half here) 4 tbsp of their cooking liquid (or water if you are using tinned chickpeas) 3 cloves of garlic, roughly chopped 150ml/¼ pint/⅔ cup good olive oil 1 tsp ground black pepper 1 tbsp tamari soy sauce or salt to your taste Juice and zest of a lemon	Put HALF of the chickpeas with the other ingredients into a goblet blender and whiz until really smooth. Add a little more water if it is a little reluctant.

. . . .

The remaining chickpeas 2 big handfuls of very fresh spinach leaves, shredded 1 big handful of fresh mint sprigs, finely chopped	Add to the crispy pitta pieces in the bowl and gently stir in the chickpea purée from the blender.

. . . .

75g/3oz silken tofu

Juice of 1 juicy lemon

1 tbsp cider vinegar

2 tbsp tahini paste

½ tsp ground black pepper

Whiz to a thick and creamy smoothness in your blender goblet. Tip the salad onto a big plate or divide between serving plates and top with the tofu 'yoghurt'.

· ·

4 tbsp pine nuts, roasted for a few minutes in a hot dry pan

Sprinkle over the salad and serve.

creamy mushroom soup

500g/1lb/5 cups mushrooms, finely sliced

25g/1oz/1 cup dried Porcini mushrooms (optional), soaked for 30 minutes in water, drained and chopped small

1 clove of garlic, sliced

1 tsp fresh thyme leaves, finely chopped (or ½ tsp dried)

2 tbsp olive oil

1 level tsp ground black pepper

Stir and sizzle over a high heat, in the bottom of a large pan, for a few minutes – the mushrooms should squeak if you have the heat high enough. Remove from heat and add...

• •

2 tbsp plain (all purpose) flour (rice or wheat)

1 tbsp vegetable bouillon powder

Stir vigorously and gently incorporate...

• •

1 litre/1¾ pints/4½ cups soya milk

Keep stirring, return to a moderate heat and bring to a gentle boil. Boil and stir for 3 minutes. Cool a little.

Whiz half the soup in your blender and return to the pan to thicken and just heat through gently.

Extra delicious when served with a couple of tiny drops of truffle oil in the bottom of each bowl.

fresh tomato soup with basil 'sour cream'

2 medium onions, chopped	Soften together gently in a heavy pan for 8–10 minutes.
3 cloves of garlic, sliced	
3 tbsp olive oil	
1 level tsp dried basil	

. . . .

1 tbsp tomato purée (paste)	Stir the tomato purée (paste) into the onions over a high heat until the oil begins to separate, 3–4 minutes. Add other ingredients to the sizzling pan, stir well and simmer over a gentle heat for about 20 minutes. Keep the lid on. Cool a little and whiz in your blender until really smooth.
6 tbsp water	
1 tbsp vegetable bouillon powder	
1 tsp runny honey (optional)	
6 big juicy tomatoes, chopped	

. . . .

Basil 'Sour Cream'

Generous handful of fresh basil (keep a few little sprigs for decoration)	Whiz until smooth in your blender. You may need to stop and scrape down the sides to keep it moving. Serve the soup hot in warm bowls with a spoonful of basil cream and a sprig of basil floating on top.
75g/3oz silken tofu	
Juice of a juicy lemon	
2 tbsp olive oil	
Pinch of black pepper	

midsummer rice salad

If you grow your own veggies, this one is even more magical.

175g/6oz/1 cup brown basmati
  rice, cooked
125g/4oz/⅔ cup fresh podded
  peas, raw
The hearts of 2 large, fresh globe
  artichokes, cooked and
  chopped (or 6 little ones from
  a jar, quartered)
2 tiny baby courgettes (zucchini),
  sliced
2 courgette (zucchini) flowers,
  shredded (optional, but if you
  have them it looks very pretty)
8 fresh mint leaves, shredded
3 tbsp good olive oil
1 tbsp tamari soy sauce
Juice from a juicy lemon
1 level tsp ground black pepper

Combine gently in a pretty salad bowl and serve. If you have used fresh artichokes, surround the salad with the pulled-off 'petals' and use to scoop!

minty tsatziki

If you can get good soya yoghurt or make your own then you can use it instead of the dressing. I always find it difficult to get hold of a sugar-free variety so I invented this alternative.

1 large cucumber, grated 1 tsp honey 4 cloves of garlic, grated	Squeeze together well and press into a sieve to drip.
175g/6oz plain tofu 2 tbsp lemon juice 1 tbsp cider vinegar 10 fresh mint leaves 1 tsp mint sauce or jelly (optional) ½ tsp ground black pepper 1 tbsp olive oil (optional)	To make the dressing, whiz together in your blender until smooth. It is quite a thick mix so you may need to stop and scrape down the sides a couple of times. Turn into a large bowl and beat in the cucumber mix. Chill to serve.

new potato and green bean salad

900g/2lb small new potatoes, scrubbed and cooked in their skins

200g/8oz/2⅔ cups French (green) beans, topped and tailed and cooked in boiling water for 8 minutes

2 tsp green peppercorns in brine (optional)

1 tbsp capers in brine (optional)

Drain and combine in a large salad bowl.

• •

1 small onion, chopped

1 clove of garlic, chopped

150ml/¼ pint/⅔ cup soya milk

4 tbsp olive oil

4 tbsp lemon juice

1 tsp runny honey

1 tsp tamari soy sauce

Whiz in your blender until you have a smooth, creamy dressing and gently mix into the salad bowl. Serve immediately while still warm or chill for later.

peanut, carrot and courgette salad

3 courgettes (zucchini), coarsely grated or cut into julienne strips (fine matchsticks)

2 medium carrots, coarsely grated or cut into julienne strips (fine matchsticks)

4 tbsp roasted peanuts (salted or not to your taste), ground or finely chopped

1 tsp honey

1 tbsp fresh mint, finely chopped

2 tbsp coriander (cilantro) leaves, finely chopped

Juice from 1 lemon

Combine in a salad bowl.

. . . .

1 tbsp olive oil

1 tsp black mustard seeds (brown)

2 tsp whole cumin seeds

½ tsp asafoetida powder (optional but very good)

1 tsp crushed dried red chilli

Heat the oil until just beginning to smoke and quickly add the spices. They will splutter madly so have a lid handy. Fry for about 1 minute and pour over the salad, mix and serve immediately.

warm barley salad

125g/4oz/½ cup barley grain	Simmer the barley in plenty of water for about 35–40 minutes until soft.

- -

1 tbsp Dijon mustard 2 cloves of garlic, crushed 4 tbsp olive oil 1 tbsp tamari soy sauce 1 tbsp cider vinegar or lemon juice 2 tbsp fresh parsley, very finely chopped Grind or two of black pepper	Whisk together in a large bowl to make the dressing.

- -

2 tbsp sesame seeds 2 tsp whole cumin seeds 1 tbsp sunflower seeds	Roast together in a dry heavy pan, shaking about to roast evenly, for a few minutes until starting to pop and smoke a little. Add to the dressing.

- -

2 carrots, grated 2 cauliflower florets, grated 1 small onion, finely chopped 10 tiny white mushrooms, finely sliced 1 sheet of nori seaweed, toasted just until the colour changes to bright green, cooled and crumbled (optional but very good!)	Stir gently into the seeds and dressing.

- -

Strain any water from the barley and tip the hot grains onto the waiting goodies, stir well and eat immediately! If you want to be really smart you can press some into a little bowl or glass that has been rubbed with olive oil, invert and turn out onto a plate, then scatter with a little more toasted nori to serve.

Try other variations of raw veggies to find your favourites. Just make sure they are all cut thinly, grated or julienned.

avocado with fresh strawberry vinaigrette

10 ripe strawberries

3 tbsp cider vinegar

6 tbsp olive oil

1 tsp honey

2 tsp raspberry vinegar (optional)

Whiz until smooth in the blender.

· ·

2 large, perfectly ripe avocados, halved and peeled

If you cut them in half and remove the stone you should be able to just score down through the skin and peel it off in two pieces. Lay one half on 4 individual plates and slice through – press down gently to fan out.

Drizzle with the dressing and serve immediately – dazzling and delicious!

main dishes

chestnut, sage and sweet squash casserole

3 tbsp olive oil

1 tbsp finely chopped fresh sage leaves (or 1 tsp dried)

1 tbsp finely chopped fresh thyme leaves (or 1 tsp dried)

5cm/2-inch stick of cinnamon

2 bay leaves

2 medium onions, roughly chopped

2 medium carrots, sliced

Heat the oil in a heavy pan, add the herbs and spice, sizzle for a moment before adding the onions and carrots. Stir well, cover and cook gently for about 8 minutes to soften the onion.

· ·

Generous 1 tbsp tomato purée (paste)

Add to the onions and increase the heat a little. Stir and sizzle for 3–4 minutes.

· ·

Sweet squash weighing approx. 900g/2lb, peeled, deseeded and cut into big bite-size chunks (butternut, kabocha, blue hubbard)

Approx. 200g/8oz/1⅓ cups cooked sweet chestnuts (available vacuum packed in cans or packets)

Stir into the pan to coat well with the mix.

· ·

Approx. 1 litre/1¾ pints/4½
 cups water
1 heaped tbsp vegetable
 bouillon powder
½ tsp ground black pepper

Stir into the pan. The liquid should cover the veggies by about 2.5cm/1 inch. Bring to the boil, reduce the heat, cover and continue to cook for about 30 minutes or until the squash and carrots are nice and soft. Remove from the heat and use a wooden spoon to press 4 or 5 pieces of squash against the side of the pan. They will thicken the sauce as you stir them through gently. Serve with a hot whole grain or creamed potatoes and a green vegetable.

creamy onion and potato hotpot

Oven temperature: 190°C/375°F/Gas Mark 5

Approx. 1kg/2½lb medium-sized, floury potatoes that have been boiled, whole, for 10 minutes, cooled in cold water and then thickly sliced (peeled if you like)

2 onions, sliced

Sprig or two of fresh or dried thyme leaves

Black pepper

Layer into a nice casserole dish with a lid. Rub a little olive oil around the inside before you start.

. . . .

175g/6oz/1 cup plain cashew nut pieces

1 litre/1¾ pints/4½ cups soya milk

4 cloves of garlic

4 tsp bouillon powder

Black pepper to taste

Pinch or two of ground nutmeg

Little bunch of snipped fresh chives, if you have them

First whiz the cashews to a fine powder in your goblet blender. You may need to stop and start and give them a little shake to encourage them. Then add the other ingredients and whiz to a cream.

Pour over the layers in the casserole, giving it a little shake down to make sure the sauce goes right to the bottom of the dish. Cover and place in a moderate oven for 35 minutes. Uncover, drizzle with olive oil and brown for about 10 more minutes.

. . . .

Vary this dish with layers of other root veggies or winter squash. Serve with green leafy vegetables and salad with a zingy dressing.

dry-spiced tuna and potato bhaji

Delicious and wonderfully quick to create.

1 medium onion, finely chopped 1 bay leaf 3 tbsp oil 2 cloves of garlic, grated	Soften together in a heavy frying pan for about 5 minutes.
2 medium potatoes, scrubbed and cut into fine matchsticks	Add to the onion, stir well, cover and continue to cook over a moderate heat for about 10 minutes.
1 level tbsp turmeric powder Pinch chilli powder 1 tsp tomato purée (paste) 1 tsp ground cumin	Stir to a thick paste with a drop or two of water. Add to the pan, increase the heat a little and stir well for a few minutes to cook the spices through, taking care not to burn them.
400g/14oz (two cans) tuna fish, drained of oil or brine 1 green chilli pepper, finely chopped (optional) 1 tbsp lemon juice or cider vinegar	Add to the pan and stir really well until the tuna is well mixed with the spices and potatoes. Keep cooking for 5–6 minutes, scraping the bottom of the pan to keep the spicy bits moving. Serve hot with plain rice or piled into baked potatoes. Lovely with Minty Tsatziki (page 159).

garlic stir-fry of mixed beansprouts with divine peanut sauce

For the sauce:

2 big cloves of garlic, chopped

2 tbsp olive oil

1 tbsp roasted sesame oil

1 chilli pepper, finely chopped (optional)

Heat together gently in a small pan (non-stick is good).

....

6 tbsp peanut butter

Juice of 2 lemons

6 tbsp water

2 tsp tamari soy sauce

1 tbsp chilli sauce or Tabasco (optional)

Stir into the pan over a gentle heat. Everything will eventually mix to a lovely smooth sauce so keep stirring. Allow to boil for a moment – add more water if it's thicker than you want or boil a little longer if it's too thin.

....

1 tbsp miso paste

Remove the pan from the heat and stir in the miso thoroughly. Keep warm. I often make double as this sauce is delicious as a dip for raw veggies or with any grain dish.

....

For the stir-fry:

2 tbsp olive oil

2 tbsp roasted sesame oil

6 cloves of garlic, finely chopped or grated

5cm/2-inch piece fresh ginger root, peeled, finely chopped or grated

1 onion, finely chopped

2 tbsp plain cashew nut pieces

Heat the oils in a wok over a high heat and throw in everything else. Toss and stir for 2–3 minutes.

....

200g/8oz mixed sprouting beans and seeds (chickpeas/garbanzo beans, mung beans, lentils, alfalfa, etc.)

Throw into the wok and toss and stir over a fierce heat for a few minutes. Serve with the sauce as soon as the sprouts are hot through but not wilted.

. . . .

Brown rice or any cooked grain is the natural accompaniment.

lentil kofta with hot and sweet sauce

200g/8oz/1 cup green or brown whole lentils, simmered in water for about 20 minutes and drained. (You can use a tin of cooked lentils but they won't have quite the same texture.)

3 tbsp gram (besan) flour

2 cloves of garlic

2 tbsp whole cumin seeds *and*

1 tbsp whole coriander (cilantro) seeds, roasted in a dry pan for a few minutes

Splash of tamari soy sauce

½ tsp ground black pepper

½ a small onion, finely chopped

Pulse together in your food processor until well mixed but not utterly smooth. Chill well.

. . . .

Olive or groundnut (peanut) oil for frying

Heat in a heavy pan. These kofta can be deep- or shallow-fried. Drop spoonfuls of the lentil mixture carefully into the hot oil. If you are shallow-frying, push down gently on the tops to flatten a little and turn once during cooking. Just do a few at a time and when they are crisp and golden, remove and keep warm to serve with the sauce.

. . . .

Hot and Sweet Sauce:

6 juicy tomatoes or one tin,
    chopped

2 dried red chilli peppers (more
    or less to your taste!)

3 tbsp runny honey

2 tbsp tamari soy sauce

1 tsp Tabasco or chilli sauce (to
    your taste)

1 tsp ground black pepper

Whiz to a smooth, runny paste in your goblet blender, pour into a heavy pan and simmer gently until reduced by about a third, stirring from time to time. You can make this sauce ahead of time and reheat or serve cold with the hot lentil kofta.

A sprinkle of fresh coriander (cilantro) is a lovely finish.

grilled bean curd kebabs with spicy bbq sauce

8 tbsp water

2 tbsp tomato purée

2 tbsp Dijon or grain mustard

3 tbsp cider vinegar

3 tbsp apple juice

1 tbsp tamari soy sauce

2 tsp runny honey (optional)

1 tsp paprika

½ tsp cayenne or chilli powder

½ tsp dolce pimienton (smoky paprika), optional but very good

Whisk together in a small pan, bring to the boil and simmer gently for 5 minutes. Leave aside to cool a little.

. . . .

Approx. 500g/1lb firm fresh bean curd (tofu), cut into 2.5cm/1-inch cubes

Approx. 5 tbsp above sauce

Combine together gently. The best way to do this is with your hands in a large bowl – messy but efficient! Thread pieces onto metal or wooden skewers, 4 or 5 on each. Carefully place on baking parchment on a plate or cookie sheet and freeze for at least one hour.

To cook – just pop kebabs (kebobs), still frozen, under a hot grill (broiler), turning as they brown. Baste with a little extra sauce until well browned and hot through. Serve with rice, the remaining sauce and a salad.

(If you want to make a lot of these for future meals just wrap them individually in clingfilm (plastic wrap), once frozen, to store.)

root ribbon pasta with wilted rocket and chilli

6 cloves of garlic, sliced

2 big parsnips, as long as you can find, peeled and stripped into 'ribbons' using a swivel-headed vegetable peeler

Put the garlic into a large pan with plenty of water, bring to the boil and drop in the parsnip ribbons. Return to the boil and drain (keep the water).

200g/8oz pasta ribbons such as tagliatelle, cooked and drained (if using wheat-free, you may have to choose spaghetti)

Add the parsnip water when cooking the pasta.

5 tbsp olive oil

1 dried red chilli pepper, crumbled

1 fresh green chilli pepper, very finely chopped

4 cloves of garlic, very finely chopped

4 stars of star anise

2 bay leaves

4 anchovies, very finely chopped (optional)

Heat the oil and sizzle together for a couple of seconds until the garlic is just beginning to turn golden. A wok is good for this part.

200g/8oz fresh rocket leaves (rucola), roughly chopped

1 tbsp tamari soy sauce (optional)

Throw into the pan and toss and stir together. Add the parsnip ribbons and pasta, mix well and heat through. Serve piping hot with a sprinkling of nutritional yeast flakes and/or snipped chives.

roasted squash, leek and bean gratin

Oven temperature: 200°C/400°F/Gas Mark 6

1 onion, finely chopped 2 bay leaves 2 tbsp olive oil 2 tbsp soya margarine	Soften together in a heavy pan over a gentle heat for about 8–10 minutes, until the onion is nice and slushy. Remove from the heat.
3 heaped tbsp organic white flour	Stir into the pan with the onions until quite smooth and well mixed.
850ml/1½ pints/3¾ cups soya milk	Gently whisk into the pan, adding a little at a time. Return to a gentle heat and stir while it comes to the boil and thickens.
1 level tsp grated nutmeg 1 tbsp bouillon powder 6 tbsp nutritional yeast flakes (or more to your taste) 1 level tsp ground black pepper	Add to the pan and simmer and stir for a few minutes. Cool for a minute or two, fish out the bay leaves and whiz with a hand blender (or in a goblet blender) until smooth.
4 or 5 medium leeks, washed, trimmed and sliced into 5cm/2-inch pieces 5 tbsp olive oil 1 squash, peeled deseeded and chopped (butternut is good) Sprig of rosemary 4 cloves of garlic, sliced	Toss together until well coated in the oil and turn into a wide, shallow casserole or ovenproof dish. Cover with the lid or foil and pop into a hot oven for 20 minutes. Uncover and bake for a few more minutes until the vegetables are just soft and browning. Remove from the oven.

500g/1lb cooked beans (use any cooked or tinned beans you have to hand. Butterbeans or flageolet work well.)

Stir gently into the vegetables and pour your creamy sauce over the top. Give the dish a little shake to settle the sauce.

To flavour:

Olive oil

Tamari soy sauce

Nutmeg

Black pepper

Drizzle and sprinkle a little of each over the top of the gratin. Bake in a moderate oven for 25 minutes or until the squash is really soft. Remove from the oven, golden and bubbling.

Lovely with a green leafy vegetable, broccoli or salad or both.

roasted vegetable and quinoa pilaf with rich piquant sauce

Oven temperature: 190°C/375°F/Gas Mark

2 medium red (bell) peppers, deseeded and chopped into chunks

1 yellow bell pepper, deseeded and chopped into chunks

½ a fresh pineapple, peeled and chopped into chunks (or a can of chunks in natural juice)

3 pink onions, chopped into chunks

1 small bulb of fennel, chopped into chunks (or 2 tsp fennel seeds or both)

5 tbsp olive oil

1 tsp honey

1 tbsp tamari soy sauce

Combine in a heavy roasting pan or casserole dish so that the veggies are well coated. Roast uncovered in a moderate oven for 45 minutes until the veggies are soft and beginning to brown. If they are browning too quickly, reduce the heat slightly.

· ·

4 cups water

500g/1lb quinoa grain

Bring the water to the boil and add the grain. Return to boiling point, reduce to a simmer, cover and cook gently for 15 minutes. Remove from the heat and place a clean cloth or some kitchen paper between the pan and the lid and set aside.

· ·

3 tbsp cider vinegar

1 tbsp balsamic vinegar

1 level tsp cayenne pepper (or
splash of sweet chilli sauce or
paprika)

1 tsp honey

1 tbsp lemon juice

Mix the ingredients by giving them a quick whiz in the blender or food processor then add about a third of the roasted vegetables. Make sure you get bits of them all in the mix. Process to a smooth or chunky sauce, as you prefer. Stir the remaining vegetables and pan juices into the quinoa, mix well and serve with the sauce. Depending on how quickly you do all this, you may find that you need to reheat the pilaf and/or sauce just before serving.

salmon nestled on leeks and watercress

4 tbsp olive oil

5 stars of star anise

3 medium leeks, washed, trimmed and cut across into pieces about 5cm/2 inches long – then each piece cut lengthways into thin strips

2 handfuls of chopped watercress

25g/1oz fresh ginger root, peeled, sliced thinly and shredded

1 tsp ground black pepper

Heat the oil in a heavy, shallow pan with a tight-fitting lid (a frying pan/skillet is fine). Throw in the star anise, give the pan a shake and add the other ingredients. Allow to sizzle over a moderate heat for about 5 minutes. Lower the heat, cover and continue to cook gently for about 8 minutes.

. . . .

10 tbsp water

4 pieces of salmon, approx. 75g/3oz each

Tamari soy sauce

Black pepper

Increase the heat a little and add the water. Place the salmon (skin side up if you have fillets) on top of the vegetables, cover again and allow to simmer gently for 10 minutes. Give the salmon a little press – it will feel firm when cooked through. You can now gently peel and discard the skin from the top of the salmon fillets with a knife. Splash the top of the fish with tamari, sprinkle with black pepper and continue cooking gently, uncovered, until most of the liquid has evaporated but the veggies are not dry. Serve piping hot with a whole-grain dish, creamed root vegetables or garlic mashed potatoes.

steam-roasted root veggies with basil

Oven temperature: 200°C/400°F/Gas Mark 6

1 medium celeriac root

1 sweet potato

1 medium parsnip

1 onion

2 large ripe tomatoes or a few sun-dried (or both)

1 medium butternut or kabocha squash, peeled, deseeded and chopped into large, bite-size chunks

3 tbsp olive oil

8 cloves of garlic, peeled and left whole

At least one handful of roughly chopped fresh basil (the more the better)

1 level tsp ground black pepper

. . . .

2 tbsp tamari soy sauce

Peel and chop the celeriac, sweet potato, parsnip, onion and tomatoes into large, bite-size chunks. Combine all the ingredients in a heavy casserole (one with a tight-fitting lid) and sizzle together over ferocious heat for about 5 minutes, stirring well. Cover tightly and place in a hot oven for 35 minutes. Remove from the oven and stir gently.

When the vegetables are good and soft splash on…

and return to the oven, uncovered, for 5 more minutes to brown a little. Serve drizzled with pesto or a squeeze of lemon, if you have some to hand.

spinach and artichoke pizza

This dough mix will make 1 large or 4 little individual pizzas.
Oven temperature: 230°C/450°F/Gas Mark 8

1 level tbsp dried yeast 230ml/8fl oz/1 cup warm water	Mix in a large bowl and leave somewhere warm for 10 minutes until frothy.

340g/12oz/2½ cups strong wholewheat flour plus extra for kneading (use a mix of brown and white bread flours if you prefer) 3 tbsp olive oil 2 tsp tamari soy sauce 1 tsp dried oregano	Mix into the frothy yeast until you have a wettish dough. Turn out onto a well-floured surface and knead and stretch until you have smooth, elastic dough. You will have to knead for at least 10 minutes, adding more flour, as it will be sticky to start with. Don't cheat on the time as this part really counts for good dough. Put the dough into an oiled bowl, cover with a damp cloth and leave in a warm place to double in size – about an hour. Tip the dough back onto a floured surface and give it a few little punches, then knead again for a few minutes. Either roll and stretch into a big circle or divide into 4 balls and roll to make smaller bases. Place on an oiled baking sheet and leave somewhere warm while you assemble your topping.

3 tbsp tomato purée (paste) 3 tbsp olive oil 1 tsp dried oregano	Whisk together in a little bowl.

2 tbsp olive oil

200g/8oz/4 cups fresh spinach
   leaves

3 cloves of garlic, thinly sliced

Heat the oil and toss the spinach and garlic over a high flame for a few minutes until wilted and softened. Remove from the heat.

200g/8oz jar of marinated
   artichoke hearts, sliced

Toss together with the spinach to coat with oil and herbs.

. . . .

6 spring onions (scallions),
   shredded

1 tbsp olive oil

Oregano, fresh or dried

Spread or brush the tomato mix over the pizza base and scatter vegetables over the top. Pop into a hot oven for about 15 minutes.

. . . .

50g/2oz plain tofu

2 tbsp olive oil

2 cloves of garlic

Black pepper to taste

4 tbsp nutritional yeast flakes

Splash of tamari soy sauce

While it's cooking:

Whiz to a cream in a goblet blender. You may need to scrape down the sides once or twice to keep it moving.

Quickly take the pizza out of the oven, blob the creamy mix on to look like slices of mozzarella cheese, and pop back in the oven for another 5–10 minutes until golden and heavenly smelling. Scatter with fresh oregano leaves if you have any and serve with salad.

tunisian-style butter beans

2 medium onions, finely chopped 4 tbsp olive oil 5cm/2-inch cinnamon stick 1 bay leaf 2 cloves of garlic, sliced 5 cloves	Soften together in a heavy pan over moderate heat for 10 minutes.

1 level tbsp ground cinnamon 1 level tsp ground nutmeg 1 tbsp tomato purée (paste) 1 tbsp tamari soy sauce 50g/2oz currants	Add to the pan and increase the heat while you stir and sizzle for 3–4 minutes.

200g/8oz/1 cup (dry weight) butter beans, cooked or 2 large tins butter beans (chickpeas/garbanzo beans work well too) Splash of cider vinegar (optional) 6 tbsp water or apple juice	Add to the pan and stir well until the butter beans are well coated. Reduce the heat, cover and simmer gently for 10 minutes. Take care that it doesn't dry out. Serve with Roasted Vegetable and Quinoa Pilaf with Rich Piquant Sauce or scoop up with wholewheat pitta breads.

puddings and cookies

almond dessert cream

200g/8oz almonds, flaked (2½ cups) or whole (1½ cups), with or without skins

Whiz in your blender to a fine powder followed by...

• •

450ml/¾ pint/2 cups soya milk or rice milk (less for a thicker cream)

Few drops of almond essence

Whiz and pour over a bowl of delicious apricots or plums braised in apple juice with a splash of maple syrup.

apricot and orange gratin

Oven temperature: 220°C/425°F/Gas Mark 7

10 large, ripe, fresh apricots	Split in half, remove stones and place skin-side down in a greased gratin dish. Try to find a dish big enough for them to fit in a single layer.
10 tsp marmalade (or sugar-free orange preserve)	Nestle ½ teaspoon in each apricot in the hole where the stone was.
200g/8oz/1½ cups almonds 1 tsp vanilla essence 1 tbsp honey 570ml/1 pint/2½ cups soya milk	Whiz in your blender until you have a thick, smooth, 'double cream' consistency – you may need a little more milk. Pour over the apricots and give the dish a little shake to settle the sauce. Bake in a hot oven for 20–25 minutes until golden and heavenly smelling. Serve warm or cold.

banana and walnut fudge torte

Oven temperature: 180°C/350°F/Gas Mark 4

150ml/¼ pint/⅔ cup apple juice concentrate 1 tbsp olive oil 3 bananas 2 tsp vanilla essence	Beat together in your food processor using the plastic blade attachment.
200g/8oz/1½ cups wholewheat (rice) flour 1 tbsp baking powder 2 heaped tsp ground cinnamon	Sift together and add to the processor.
125g/4oz/1 cup chopped walnuts	Add to the processor and pulse a few times to quickly form a soft batter. Pour half into a greased cake tin.
2 tbsp walnuts, chopped 1 tbsp ground cinnamon	Mix together and sprinkle half over the cake mix in the tin. Top with the rest of the banana mixture (work quickly) and then sprinkle the remaining nuts and cinnamon on the top. Place in a moderate oven for about 25 minutes. Cool before serving.

figs baked in lemon cream

Oven temperature: 200°C/400°F/Gas Mark 6

500g/1lb/3 cups dried figs (or
  semi-dried or honey-dried)
2 tsp vanilla essence
Apple juice to cover

Soak figs overnight until plump and soft. Cut figs in half and use to cover the bottom of a lightly greased gratin dish.

200ml/7fl oz/¾ cup pineapple
  juice
3 tbsp cornflour (cornstarch)
4 tbsp water

Bring the pineapple juice to the boil. Blend the cornflour (cornstarch) to a really smooth, runny paste with the water and pour into the boiling pineapple juice, whisking vigorously. Boil and stir for a couple of minutes and remove from heat.

1 large banana
Juice from a juicy lemon
Zest of 1 lemon
Splash of soya milk

Whiz in the blender until smooth and runny. Whisk into the hot pineapple pan and pour over the figs. Bake in a hot oven for 15 minutes until browned. Chill to serve.

raspberry cream pie

Oven temperature: 190°C/375°F/Gas Mark 5

125g/4oz/scant cup whole-wheat flour 75g/3oz/½ cup fine or medium oatmeal 1 tbsp tahini 50g/2oz/¼ cup soya margarine 2 tbsp olive oil	Rub in as for pastry.

· ·

1 tbsp malt extract	Stir into the mix to form a crumbly pastry – you may need a drop or two of water. Press the mixture into a flan dish or tin to make a pastry shell and bake for 20 minutes.

· ·

200g/8oz/2 cups raspberries (fresh or frozen)	Scatter *half* the raspberries over the cooked and cooled pastry...

· ·

Remaining raspberries Splash of soya milk 200g/7oz silken tofu 1 tbsp arrowroot 1 banana 2 tbsp honey (or sugar) 1 tsp vanilla essence	and put the rest with all the other ingredients into your blender and whiz until smooth – the mixture should be quite thick so you may need to stop the blender and scrape down the sides. Pour the mix over the raspberries, return to the oven and bake for 30 minutes. Chill to serve.

peanut butter cookies

Oven temperature: 180°C/350°F/Gas Mark 4

150g/5oz peanut butter (crunchy or smooth but no added sugar)
50g/2oz/¼ cup soya margarine
75g/3oz/¼ cup honey
1 tsp vanilla essence

Blend to a cream in your food processor with the plastic blade attachment.

. . . .

125g/4oz/scant cup rice flour (or unbleached white wheat flour)
1 tsp baking powder

Sieve together and add to the processor. Whiz to blend quickly, stop as soon as well mixed and turn the dough out onto a lightly floured surface. Knead for a minute or two and press together.

Take large walnut-size pieces of dough and roughly roll into balls. Place well spaced on a cookie sheet and press into 'cookie' shapes with a fork. Bake in a moderate oven for 10 minutes. Allow to cool and crisp up on the cookie sheet before eating or storing.

better chocolate cake

Oven temperature: 180°C/350°F/Gas Mark 4

50g/2oz/2½ cups dried dates 200ml/7fl oz/¾ cup water	Bring to the boil, simmer for 5 minutes and cool a little.
2 tbsp flax seeds or linseeds	Whiz to a fine powder in your blender.
115ml/4fl oz/½ cup water	Add to the blender and whiz again until well mixed and frothy.
The cooked dates 175g/6oz silken or fresh tofu 2 tsp vanilla essence 1 tbsp oil 200ml/7fl oz/¾ cup maple syrup	Add to the blender and whiz until smooth.
Generous 200g/8oz/1½ cups unbleached white flour 90g/3½oz/scant cup cocoa or carob powder 1 heaped tbsp baking powder	Sieve into a large bowl and quickly beat in the blended mixture. Turn into a cake tin (approx. 25 × 3.5cm/10 × 1½ inches deep) and bake for about 25 minutes. Cool in the tin. This cake keeps well in an airtight container. For extra luxury, it can be topped with melted dark chocolate or the following rich 'cream'.

Rich Cream Topping:

75g/3oz/½ cup plain cashew nuts	Grind to a fine powder in blender then...
Approx. 4 tbsp water 125g/4oz silken tofu 3 tbsp maple syrup or honey	Add to the blender and whiz to a smooth, thick cream. Chill before using to fill or top the cake.

Variations on this cream are easy and delicious. Try adding:

3 tbsp light tahini

or

3 tbsp melted carob drops and

1 tsp vanilla essence

or

3 tbsp cocoa powder

sticky date and chocolate brownies

Oven temperature: 200°C/400°F/Gas Mark 6

200g/8oz/1½ cups stoned dates
(soft dried ones work best)
200g/8oz/1½ cups raisins
425ml/¾ pint/2 cups boiling
water

Cook together for about 5 minutes.

175g/6oz/1½ cups cocoa or
carob powder

Blend into the date mixture.

90ml/3fl oz/⅓ cup soya milk
2 tsp vanilla essence
2 tbsp olive oil
2 tbsp molasses or date syrup
½ tsp cider vinegar

Stir into the dates and mix thoroughly.

340g/12oz/2½ cups whole-
wheat flour (rice flour)
2 tsp baking powder

Sift together and quickly mix with the
date mixture. Pour into a shallow cookie
or roasting tin and bake for about
10–15 minutes. Cool in the tin and
cut into small squares to serve.

appendix 1: reference notes

CHAPTER 3 – INTOLERANCE TO DAIRY PROTEIN

1. A food allergy involves an IgE mediated reaction whereas a food intolerance involves an IgG mediated reaction.
2. Dohan, F.C. et al. 'Relapsed schizophrenics. More rapid improvement on a milk and cereal-free diet', *British Journal of Psychiatry*, 1969, 115, 595.
3. Reichelt, K. et al. 'Gluten, milk proteins and autism: dietary intervention effects on behavior and peptide secretions', *Journal of Applied Nutrition*, 1990, 42, 1–11.
4. Brostoff, J. and Gamlin, L. *The complete guide to food allergy and intolerance*, Bloomsbury, London, 1992.

CHAPTER 4 – OTHER RELATIONSHIPS BETWEEN DAIRY AND HEALTH

1. Artaud-Wild, S.M. et al. 'Differences in coronary mortality can be explained by differences in cholesterol and saturated fat intakes in 40 countries but not in France and Finland. A paradox', *Circulation*, 1993, 88, 2771–2779.
2. Chan, J.M. et al. 'Dairy products, calcium and prostate cancer risk in the Physicians' Health Study', *American Journal of Clinical Nutrition*, 2001, 74, 4, 549–554.
3. Giovannucci, E. 'Diet, 1,25(OH)$_2$ vitamin D and prostate cancer: a hypothesis', *Cancer Causes Control*, 1998, 9, 567–83.
4. Muntoni, S. et al. 'Nutritional factors and worldwide incidence of childhood type 1 diabetes', *American Journal of Clinical Nutrition*, 2000, 71, 6, 1525–1529.
5. Dahl-Jorgenson, K. et al. 'Relationship between cows' milk consumption and incidence of IDDM in childhood', *Diabetes Care*, 1991, 14, 11, 1081–1083.

6. Virtanen, S.M. et al. 'Early introduction of dairy products associated with increased risk of IDDM in Finnish children. The Childhood in Diabetes in Finland Study Group', *Diabetes*, 1993, 42, 12, 1786–1790.

7. Hegsted, D.M. 'Fractures, calcium and the modern diet', *American Journal of Clinical Nutrition*, 2001, 74, 5, 571–573.

8. Feskanich, D. et al. 'Milk, dietary calcium, and bone fractures in women: a 12-year prospective study', *American Journal of Public Health*, 1997, 87, 6, 992–997.

9. Owusu, W. et al. 'Calcium intake and the incidence of forearm and hip fractures among men', *The Journal of Nutrition*, 1997, 127, 9, 1782–1787.

10. Weinsier, R.L. and Krumdieck, C.L. 'Dairy foods and bone health: examination of the evidence', *American Journal of Clinical Nutrition*, 2000, 72, 3, 681–689.

11. Weinsier, R.L. and Krumdieck, C.L. Ibid.

12. Sesink, A.L. et al. 'Red meat and colon cancer: dietary haem-induced colonic cytotoxicity and epithelial hyperproliferation are inhibited by calcium', *Carcinogenesis*, 2001, 22, 10, 1653–1659.

13. Jiang, J. et al. 'Relation between the intake of milk fat and the occurrence of conjugated linoleic acid in human adipose tissue', *American Journal of Clinical Nutrition*, 1999, 70, 1, 21–27.

CHAPTER 5 – THE BENEFITS OF GOING ALKALINE

1. Potential Renal Acid Load chart derived from Remer, T. and Manz, F. as presented in Barzel, U.S. and Massey, L.K. 'Excess dietary protein can adversely affect bone', *The Journal of Nutrition*, 1998, 128, 6, 1051–1053.

CHAPTER 7 – FOODS TO EAT

1. Messina, M.J. 'Legumes and soybeans: overview of their nutritional profiles and health effects', *American Journal of Clinical Nutrition*, 1999, 70, 3, 439S–450S.

CHAPTER 10 – WHAT NEXT?

1. Bengmark, S. 'Ecological control of the gastrointestinal tract. The role of probiotic flora', *Gut*, 1998, 42, 2–7.
2. O'Farrelly, C. 'Just how inflamed is the normal gut?', *Gut*, 1998, 42, 603–604.
3. Collins, M.D. and Gibson, G.R. 'Probiotics, prebiotics, and synbiotics: approaches for modulating the microbial ecology of the gut', *American Journal of Clinical Nutrition*, 1999, 69, 5, 1052S–1057S.
4. Isolauri, E, et al. 'Probiotics: effects on immunity', *American Journal of Clinical Nutrition*, 2001, 73, 444S–450S.
5. Sütas, Y. et al. 'Suppression of lymphocyte proliferation in vitro by bovine caseins hydrolysed with *Lactobacillus* GG-derived enzymes', *Journal of Allergy and Clinical Immunology*, 1996, 98, 216–224.
6. Isolauri, E. et al. 'Probiotics in the management of atopic eczema', *Clin Exp Allergy*, 2000, 30,1605–1610.
7. Gibson, G.R. et al. 'Selective stimulation of bifidobacteria in the human colon by oligofructose and inulin', *Gastroenterology*, 1995, 108, 975–982.
8. Roberfroid, M.B. 'Prebiotics: preferential substrates for specific germs?', *American Journal of Clinical Nutrition*, 2001, 73, 2, 406S–409S.
9. Jensen-Jarolin, E. et al. 'Hot spices influence permeability of human intestinal epithelial monolayers', *Journal of Nutrition*, 1998, 128, 3, 577–581.
10. Brostoff, J. and Gamlin, L. *The complete guide to food allergy and intolerance*, Bloomsbury, London, 1992.

CHAPTER 11 – WHY FATS ARE ESSENTIAL

1. Kris-Etherton, P.M. et al. 'Polyunsaturated fatty acids in the food chain in the United States', *American Journal of Clinical Nutrition*, 2000, 71, 1, 179–188.
2. Ascherio, A. and Willett, W.C. 'Health effects of trans fatty acids', *American Journal of Clinical Nutrition*, 1997, 66, 1006S–1010S.
3. Salmeron, J. et al. 'Dietary fat intake and risk of type 2 diabetes in women', *American Journal of Clinical Nutrition*, 2001, 73, 6, 1019–1026.

CHAPTER 12 – FOOD INTOLERANCE AND WEIGHT LOSS

1. Glycaemic Index chart derived from Foster-Powell, K. et al. 'International table of glycemic index and glycemic load values: 2002', *American Journal of Clinical Nutrition*, 2002, 76, 1, 5–56.

2. Jenkins, D.J. et al. 'Glycemic index: overview of implications in health and disease', *American Journal of Clinical Nutrition*, 2002, 76, 1, 266S–273S.

CHAPTER 13 – CALCIUM AND OTHER IMPORTANT NUTRIENTS

1. Weinsier, R.L. and Krumdieck, C.L. 'Dairy foods and bone health: examination of the evidence', *American Journal of Clinical Nutrition*, 2000, 72, 3, 681–689.

2. Seelig, M.S. 'Interrelationship of magnesium and estrogen in cardiovascular and bone disorders, eclampsia, migraine and premenstrual syndrome', *Journal of American Coll Nutrition*, 1993, 12, 4, 442–458.

3. Passwater, R.A. and Cranton, E.M. *Trace elements, hair analysis and nutrition*, Keats Publishing, 1983.

4. Abraham, G.E. and Grewal, H. 'A total dietary program emphasizing magnesium instead of calcium. Effect on the mineral density of calcaneous bone in postmenopausal women on hormonal therapy', *Journal of Reproductive Medicine*, 1990, 35, 5, 503–507.

5. Dimai, H.P. et al. 'Daily oral magnesium supplementation suppresses bone turnover in young adult males', *Journal of Clinical Endocrinology and Metabolism*, 1998, 83, 8, 2742–2748.

6. Liu, C.C. et al. 'Magnesium directly stimulates osteblast proliferation', *Journal of Bone and Mineral Research*, 1988, 3, S104.

7. Cohen, L. and Kitzes, R. 'Infrared spectroscopy and magnesium content of bone mineral in osteoporotic women', *Israel Journal of Medical Science*, 1981, 17, 12, 1123–1125.

8. Tranquilli, A.L. et al. 'Calcium, phosphorus, and magnesium intakes correlate with bone mineral content in postmenopausal women', *Gynecology Endocrinology*, 1994, 8, 55–58.

9. Sojka, J.E. and Weaver, C.M. 'Magnesium supplementation and osteoporosis', *Nutrition Review*, 1995, 53, 3, 71–74.

10. Stendig-Lindberg, G. et al. 'Trabecular bone density in a two year controlled trial of peroral magnesium in osteoporosis', *Magnesium Research*, 1993, 6, 155–163.

11. Feskanich, D. et al. 'Vitamin K intake and hip fractures in women: a prospective study', *American Journal of Clinical Nutrition*, 1999, 69, 1, 74–79.

CHAPTER 14 – BEYOND CALCIUM – HOW TO LOOK AFTER YOUR BONES

1. Nordin, B.E.C. et al. 'The problem of calcium requirement', *American Journal of Clinical Nutrition*, 1987, 45, 1295–1304.

2. World Health Organization Press Release, 'Bone Health: Organizations and individuals must act now to avoid an impending epidemic', 1999, number 68.

3. Massey, L.K. 'Does excess dietary protein adversely affect bone? Symposium overview', *Journal of Nutrition*, 1998, 128, 1048–1050.

4. Krieger, N.S. et al. 'Acidosis inhibits osteoblastic and stimulates osteoclastic activity in vitro', *American Journal of Physiology*, 1992, 262, F442–448.

5. Frassetto, L.A. et al. 'Worldwide incidence of hip fracture in elderly women: relation to consumption of animal and vegetables foods', *Journals of Gerontology Series A: Biological Sciences and Medical Sciences*, 2000, 55, M585–592.

6. New, S.A. et al. 'Dietary influences on bone mass and bone metabolism: further evidence of a positive link between fruit and vegetable consumption and bone health?', *American Journal of Clinical Nutrition*, 2000, 71, 1, 142–151.

7. Weaver, C.M. et al. 'Choices for achieving adequate dietary calcium with a vegetarian diet', *American Journal of Clinical Nutrition*, 1999, 70, 3, 543S–548S.

8. Berkelhammer, C.H. et al. 'Acetate and hypercalciuria during total parenteral nutrition', *American Journal of Clinical Nutrition*, 1988, 48, 1482–1486.

9. Heaney, R.P. et al. 'Absorbability of calcium from brassica vegetables: broccoli, bok choy, and kale', *Journal of Food Science*, 1993, 58, 1378–1380.

10. Greger, J.L. 'Nondigestible carbohydrates and mineral bioavailability', *Journal of Nutrition*, 1999, 129, 1434S–1435S.

11. Felson, D.T. 'Alcohol intake and bone mineral density in elderly men and women', *American Journal of Epidemiology*, 1995, 142, 485–492.

12. Wolf, R.L. et al. 'Factors associated with calcium absorption efficiency in pre- and perimenopausal women', *American Journal of Clinical Nutrition*, 2000, 72, 2, 466–471.

13. Barzel, U.S. and Massey, L.K. 'Excess dietary protein can adversely affect bone', *Journal of Nutrition*, 1998, 128, 6, 1051–1053.
14. Hopper, J.L. and Seeman, E. 'The bone density of female twins discordant for tobacco use', *New England Journal of Medicine*, 1994, 330, 6, 387–392.
15. Michaelson, D. et al. 'Bone Mineral Density in Women with Depression', *New England Journal of Medicine*, 1996, 335, 1176–81.

CHAPTER 15 – SIDE-EFFECTS OF MODERN DAIRY FARMING

1. The *Guardian* newspaper, 7 September 1999.
2. Hoskins, R. and Lobstein, T. 'The perfect pinta? A look at the environmental and social effects of dairy production', *Food Facts No 2*, 1999, from *Sustainable Agriculture, Food and Environment*.
3. Organic Milk Producers Association, 2001.
4. 'Dioxins and PCBs in retail cows' milk in England', Food Surveillance Information Sheet Number 136, Ministry of Agriculture Fisheries and Food, December 1997.
5. Santillo, D., Stringer, R.L. and Johnston, P.A. 'The global distribution of PCBs, organochlorine pesticides, polychlorinated dibenzo-p-dioxins and polychlorinated dibenzofurans using butter as an integrative matrix', 2000, Greenpeace Research Laboratories Technical Note.
6. The Organic Milk Producers Association, 2001.
7. The Food Commission Press Release, 23 July 1996.
8. 'Annual Report of the Working Party on Pesticide Residues', 1996, MAFF Health and Safety Executive.
9. 'Dioxins and their effects on human health', Fact Sheet number 225, 1999, World Health Organization.

CHAPTER 16 – FURTHER INFORMATION

1. Hollox E.J. et al. 'Lactase haplotype diversity in the old world', *American Journal of Human Genetics*, 2001, 68, 160–172.
2. National Institute of Health.
3. Chart derived from data from the National Institute of Health and the American Gastroenterology Association.

4. Grant, W.B. 'Milk and other dietary influences on coronary heart disease', *Alternative Medical Review*, 1998, 3, 4, 281–294.

5. Grant, W.B. 'Lactose maldigestion and calcium from dairy products', *American Journal of Clinical Nutrition*, 1999, 70, 2, 301A–302.

6. Horrobin, D.F. 'Essential fatty acid metabolism and its modification in atopic eczema', *American Journal of Clinical Nutrition*, 2000, 71, 1, 367S–372S.

appendix 2: foods that contain dairy

Look out for the following terms on the labels of processed foods:

Whey
Milk solids
Casein
Sodium caseinate
Lactose
Sodium lactylate
Lactalbumin
Galactose

Here is a list of foods that contain dairy:

Bread and bread products
Butter
Buttermilk
Cakes
Cheese
Chocolate
Cookies
Cow's milk
Cream
Crêpes
Custard
Fromage frais
Frozen yoghurt

Ice cream
Instant mashed potato
Instant milk-based drinks (hot chocolate, Ovaltine, etc.)
Meat, processed (casein) (not in Kosher foods)
Mousse
Muffins
Pancakes
Pizza
Powdered milk
Puddings
Quiche
Rice 'cheese'
Sauces
Soups
Vegetable spreads
Yoghurt

hidden sources of dairy or lactose

Note: minute amounts of lactose are only a problem for those with extreme lactose intolerance. Do not stop taking medication without consulting your doctor first.

Non-dairy creams
Non-dairy whipped toppings
Prescription drugs (lactose)
Other medication (lactose)

appendix 3: shopping list

dairy substitutes

Soya milk
Rice milk
Oat milk
Soya cream
Soya yoghurt (live)

healing foods

Flax seeds
Fresh pineapple
Fresh ginger root or dried ginger tea
Cruciferous vegetables (e.g. broccoli, cauliflower, cabbage, kale,
   Brussels sprouts)
Onions and garlic
Black cherries and blueberries

supplements

Dairy-free probiotic supplement
Evening primrose oil (1,500mg per day) or GLA (150mg per day)
Omega-3 fish oils (if you don't eat oily fish)
A good multivitamin

A good multimineral
Vitamin C supplement (500–1,000mg per day)
FOS powder (stage two)
Glutamine powder (stage two)

appendix 4: calcium content of various foods[1]

	Serving Size	Calcium Content (mg)
Fish		
Salmon	170g/6oz	440
Sardines	170g/6oz	620
Shrimp	170g/6oz	220
Trout	170g/6oz	384
Tuna	170g/6oz	20
FRUIT AND VEGETABLES		
Apple	1 medium	10
Banana	1 medium	8
Bok choy	55g/2oz	79
Broccoli	85g/3oz	50
Brussels sprouts	85g/3oz	40
Cabbage, red	85g/3oz	48
Cabbage, white	85g/3oz	40
Cauliflower	1 cup	34
Chinese cabbage greens	55g/2oz	239
Chinese mustard greens	55g/2oz	212
Collard greens	1 cup	357
Courgette (zucchini)	85g/3oz	16
Figs, dried or fresh	5 medium	135
Grapefruit	1 medium	30
Kale	55g/2oz	61
Lettuce	30g/1oz	10

	Serving Size	Calcium Content (mg)
FRUIT AND VEGETABLES (CONT.)		
Okra	85g/3oz	63
Orange	1 medium	50
Parsley	30g/1oz	30
Potato	1 medium	20
Seaweed – kombu	85g/3oz	168
Seaweed – nori	85g/3oz	70
Seaweed – wakame	85g/3oz	150
Sweet potato	1 medium	44
Turnip greens	1 cup	198
Watercress	85g/3oz	120
SOYA PRODUCTS		
Soya milk, fortified	300ml/½ pint	360
Soya milk, unfortified	300ml/½ pint	80
Soya yoghurt	85g/3oz	125
Tofu, firm, calcium-fortified	115g/4oz	258
Tofu, medium, calcium-fortified	115g/4oz	130
NUTS AND SEEDS		
Almond butter	1 tablespoon	43
Almonds	30g/1oz	80
Brazil nuts	30g/1oz	52
Flax seeds	30g/1oz	64
Hazelnuts	30g/1oz	56
Pistachio nuts	30g/1oz	40
Sesame seeds, hulled	30g/1oz	45
Sesame seeds, unhulled	30g/1oz	290
Sunflower seeds	30g/1oz	34
Tahini	1 tablespoon	64
Walnuts	30g/1oz	31

	Serving Size	**Calcium Content (mg)**
BEANS		
Pinto	115g/4oz	40
Red	115g/4oz	40
White	115g/4oz	113
FLUIDS		
Goat's milk, enriched	300ml/½ pint	300
Orange juice, calcium-fortified	300ml/½ pint	320
Orange juice, fresh	300ml/½ pint	27
Rice milk, calcium-enriched	300ml/½ pint	360
OTHER		
Blackstrap molasses	1 tablespoon	171

1. Chart derived from data from National Institute Health, The USDA Nutrient Data Base and other sources.

appendix 5: useful information and addresses

Dawn Hamilton and Associates

Suite 14035

Muswell Hill Broadway

London N10 2WB

Telephone: (020) 8883 2408

Email: health@drdawn.co.uk

Website: www.drdawn.co.uk

Jane Sen

www.JaneSen.com

Videos by Jane Sen available from www.JaneSen.com:

Healing Foods – Delicious and Dairy Free

Healing Foods – Juicing and Raw Power

Healing Foods – Sweet but Unrefined

finding a nutritionist

A nutritionist can arrange tests for food intolerance and gut permeability, and develop a tailor-made nutritional and eating plan suitable for your needs. Contact:

Dawn Hamilton (details above)

The Institute for Optimum Nutrition (ION)
Blades Court
Deodar Road
London SW15 2NU
Telephone: (020) 8877 9993

Send an SAE with a cheque for £2 to receive the directory of qualified nutritionists.

British Association of Nutritional Therapists (BANT)
27 Old Gloucester Street
London WC1N 3XX
Telephone: (0870) 606 1284

Send an A4 SAE with 72p of stamps for a directory of qualified nutritionists. A voluntary donation of £2 is suggested to cover costs.

intolerance testing and other tests

ELISA test
York Laboratories
In the UK: (01904) 410410 and at www.allergy-testing.com
In the USA: 1–888–751–3388 and at www.yorkallergyusa.com

Gut Permeability Test

Biolab

9 Weymouth Street

London W1N 3FF

(020) 7636 5959

Urine Peptide Test

Great Plains Laboratory

1–913–341–8949 and at www.greatplainslaboratory.com

nutritional supplements

Biocare Ltd

180 Lifford Lane

Birmingham B30 3NU

Telephone: (0121) 433 3727

Biocare offers an extensive range of supplements, including an excellent selection of intestinal support products such as probiotics, FOS and glutamine (*Permatrol*). Mail order is available or phone to get details of your nearest stockist.

Higher Nature

Burwash Common

East Sussex TN19 7LX

Telephone: (01435) 882880

Higher Nature produces *True Food Form* vitamin and mineral supplements that are better absorbed than many other supplements. They also offer probiotics, FOS and glutamine (in powder form). *The Omega Nutrition* range of essential fatty acids (in liquid or capsule form) is excellent. Higher Nature products are sold in most health-food stores. They also offer a mail-order service and will send you a free catalogue.

Solgar Vitamins
Tring
Herts HP23 5PT
Telephone: (01442) 890355

Solgar offers an extensive range of products, including three excellent multivitamin supplements (*VM75*, *VM2000* and *Omnium*). They also offer probiotics, FOS and glutamine plus a complete range of vitamin and mineral supplements and many good herbal products. Solgar products are sold in most health-food stores. Phone for details of your nearest stockist.

home care products

The Healthy House
Cold Harbour
Ruscombe
Stroud
Gloucestershire GL6 6DA
Telephone: (01453) 752216

This company specializes in allergy-free home-care products such as cleaning aids, air purifiers, water distillers and bedding. Phone for a free catalogue.

index